The Code of Love

The Code of Life

Communications
&
System of Health

Yuri Spilny

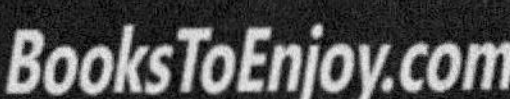

BooksToEnjoy.com
Yuri's Hill
Peppermint Meadow, HC1, Box 106
Kernville, CA 93238

The Code of Life Communications & System of Health
The Code of Love

Copyright © 2019 Yuri Spilny

For information related to the book, contact
yuri@bookstoenjoy.com
or
Editor Katya Khellblau
kat.khell@gmail.com

ISBN: 9798553643324

United States Copyright Office
Registration number TX 8-949-744

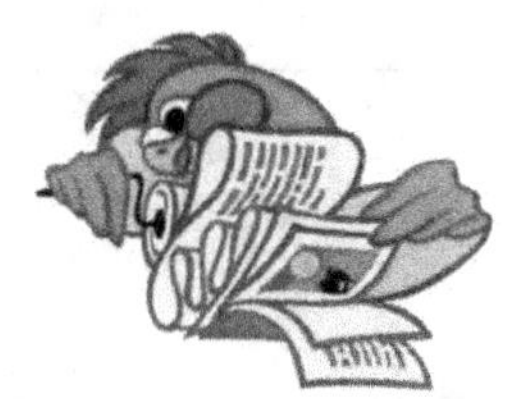

BooksToEnjoy.com

To my beautiful parents,

Gregory and Anna

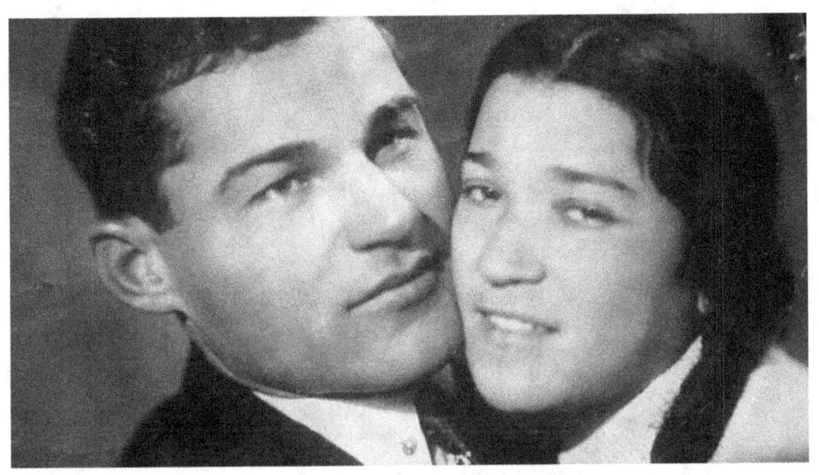

I am Forever Grateful

...Love is infinite, as the stars have no number and the sea no
rest.   From: *Gates of the Dead*

Smile today, forget tomorrow,
For tomorrow may call the clouds and sorrow.
Enjoy the rose while it's fragrant and fresh.
Enjoy the mellow melody while it sings
The silent love of the Infinite today.
For yesterday is gone, and tomorrow may delay,
Or it may never come.
Yes, while laughter bubbles at thy door,
Drink from that fount evermore,
For tomorrow the spring may dry,
And its solacing voice may die.
Drink, drink, drink the wine of laughter today,
Burn, burn, burn your fears of all tomorrows and
yesterday.
Life is a dewdrop perched on the grassy blade of time,
Trembling to fly with the sun's rays and end this strife.
Catch the dewdrop and ride on its wings,
On to the shores where eternity sings.

Yesterday and tomorrow are unseen strips far away.
Fly to thy Freedom, fly from thy prison
in the ark of a sunny day!

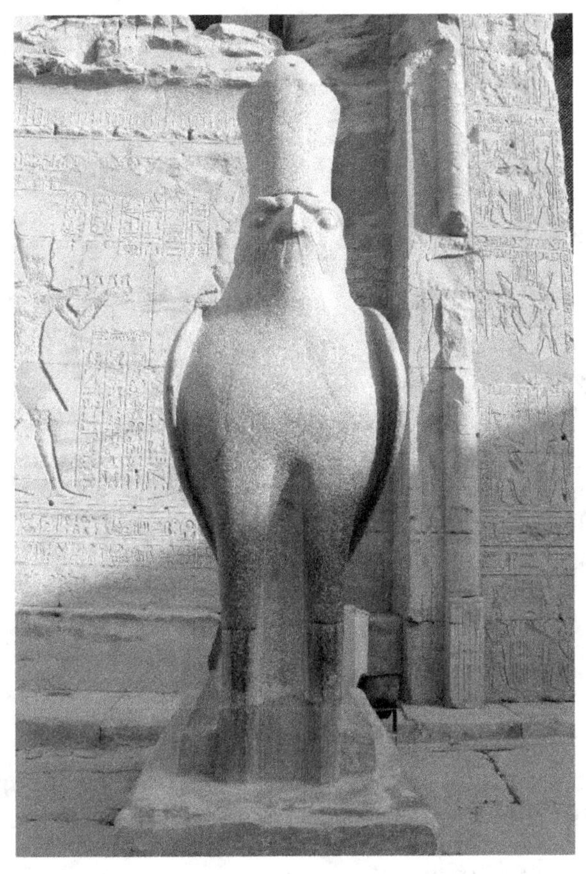

Images of Horus and The Tree of Life are Egypt's most valuable contributions to humanity. Read the Chapter *Fountain of Youth: The Code of Horus with the Tree of Life.*

Contents

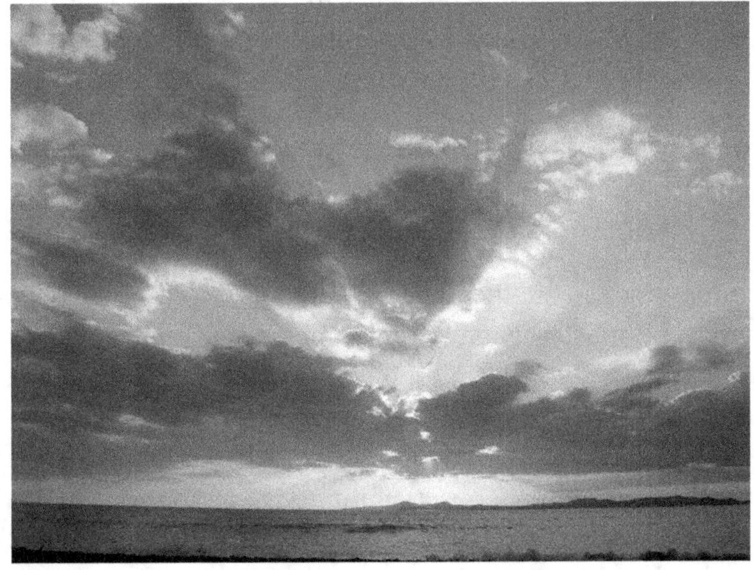

Ah, Love! Could thou and I, with Fate conspire.
To grasp the sorry Scheme of Things entire,
Would not we shatter it to bits – and then
Re-mold it nearer to the Heart Desire!

Introduction

"What I will reveal now to transmit to mankind will surely collide with the misunderstanding and prejudice in the world." Albert Einstein said it regarding his view of the Universal force of Love; it also applies to *The Code of life Communications and System of Health: The Code of Love.*

There is a simple and effective way to get rid of illness without the help of a doctor and medication. The method is *The Code of Life.* We have hundreds of people successfully using The Code while avoiding the doctors with their prescriptions of drugs loaded with dangerous side effects. In its free state, *The Code of Life* generates 100% energy with a frequency of 10 to the 56 power – the energy and frequency of true Love. With this benevolent power, we destroy pathogens, dissolve deposits in vessel dissolve stones, restore tissue, organs, and systems, and perform all tests and diagnoses. Thus, we become our best and only doctors.

Informatics is another inimitable application of *The Code of Life,* the most accurate communications system. It provides information on any person and subject, past and present, validating any document and event via tapping into the *Infinite Intelligence,* also the Infinite field of Knowledge. We also get instant data observability, stay on top of data quality, and detect fake data before it hurts us. We become our best and only teachers.

The decision to become your best and only doctor and teacher will start a transformation process. Right now, your mind contains tons of information that filters your every decision, often distorting your choices and thoughts. This acquired information must go except the professional knowledge necessary to do the job.

Whether it is an eastern or western spiritual and religious teaching, military or political views, or cultural beliefs, it is a hindrance.

Believe not because some old manuscripts are produced, believe not because it is your national belief, believe not because you have been made to believe from your childhood, but reason truth out with Love. If you find it will do good to one and all, believe it, live up to it, and help others live up to it.

You are conditioned to believe it is necessary to depend on something and someone. However, we are born self-sufficient and independent; nothing from the outside is required to be our best and only teachers and doctors. All data we need must come from within, connected to Infinite Intelligence.

The countless applications of *The Code of Life* include purification of water, decontamination of foodstuff, verification of the quality of the product, whether it is an automobile or honey, validation of our decisions, whether financial, relationships' or any other, and more.

You can verify that *The Code* is real by giving it to your relatives or anyone with hand arthritis and be convinced: indeed, within less than ten days, *The Code* eliminates arthritis. We would be happy to provide *The Code* and instructions upon request. Why arthritis? Because it is an excellent example of *The Code's* energy eliminating it in a short time.

The Code of Life is at the core of Life. We did not create it. It existed forever. It was hidden behind dense drop-curtain – the confusion of doctors, teachers, teachings, and misinformation. *The Code* came forth on its own when the curtain was lifted.

The Code of Life is the only way to freedom. It may sound pompous, but as you read the book, you will realize that being your best teacher and doctor is the only way to know the Truth.

Freedom means freedom from all teachers, teachings, concepts, dogmas, and beliefs. I have searched for almost 40 years like you and millions of others. The search resulted in several books with realizations that have been helpful to many people in daily life.

Only when I realized the importance of being my best and only teacher when I became my only teacher did I discover *The Code of Life*. I was 80 years old. I was not free, but a high Intel-Star (soul) energy level enabled me to discover *The Code*.

If I were free, I would discover nothing because when enlightened, one does not make discoveries; he leaves behind no traces like Buddha. Are you a searcher? Did you achieve anything with your search? Did you meet anyone who has achieved anything with their search? If you believe they did, send me this person's picture, and if it is true, I will send you $100. However, no people have experienced inner growth with their search, practices, or anything else.

It cannot be because the world spiritual industry is a ruse created by unaware self-appointed teachers with an overall Intel-Star energy level below 20%, which is a fraud. To make helpful teaching, one must have 200% energy of enlightenment. But enlightened people create nothing because they know people must discover their inner treasures. It is a seeming paradox, but only for a deficient in energy person. There are no helpful teachings because there is nothing to teach. Our inner world is already perfect, and the secret of inner growth is that we must discover this perfection.

Even this book is optional. I wrote it to help you drop all books, teachers, doctors, and medicaments. At 84, as I translated *The Code* into Russian, I had a 187% Intel-Star energy level and 167 IQ. (Freedom is 200%, as explained in the following chapter.) In this state, I saw the world and people as they were. Secrets and puzzles no longer exist for me, and history became an open book of fairytales.

Buddha was still enlightened. If enlightened, he would not follow "spiritual" traditions for twenty-four years until he realized all traditions, teachings, practices, and methods were useless. *The Code of Life Communications and System of Health* will help you cut off your fruitless search, for the search brings you nowhere. You will find the Truth only when you abandon the entire "spiritual" trash and become your best and only teacher, for the trash has been created to take you away from yourself.

Only 4% of trash separated Buddha's mind from being stark naked. A human mind cannot be 100% stark naked. An average person's mind has 75% rubbish, separating it from being stark naked.

Indian spiritual folks and Buddhists' overall Intel-Star energy level is 7%. Fraud is inevitable at 28%. For millenniums, Indian spiritual people and Buddhists have perpetuated lies and spread them worldwide.

As the East describes it, the life of the Buddha is a big lie fabricated by the Buddhists. His father was a poor carpenter, not a king. Buddha left his family when he was 16. He searched for 24 long years until he realized the futility of the search.

It is a paradox, for why who is free would not help others to freedom? This question could be answered only by the free one. After he was free, Buddha never said a word, did not heal anyone, and left no traces.

"When a student is ready, the teacher appears." The "teachers" have crafted many similar expressions to deceive you and promote themselves. Words are meaningless unless they suggest the right action. The Truth is that when a student is ready, all teachers disappear together with teachings, books, seminars, and retreats. No teachers know anything, as there is nothing to know, nothing to teach, nothing to learn, and nowhere to reach. Still, a great deception entices people, pushing them to search and search and never find anything except far away stripes of yesterdays and tomorrow glimmering in the darkness of the illusion of the possible.

Look into your heart and ask yourself: "in truth, did I find anything with my search?" If you are honest, the answer will be "NO! I got nothing from my search." Nobody did. "Helped" by the "teachers" and gurus claiming to be enlightened with their deficient energy levels, people are forcing themselves into ignorant beliefs. When you discard all "spiritual" nonsense and become your best and only teacher, your brain's receptors will open to information from the *Infinite Intelligence* that will guide you like it is guiding every life in nature. Only then will you find the Truth?

With *The Code of Life,* you can verify past and present spiritual information and realize there is no truth in it. You will see there are no enlightened people in the world. Every teacher is a windbag. All so-called Buddha's saying, writings, teachings, and techniques are deception created by the ignorant followers, for Buddha wrote nothing. He was illiterate. Buddha was teaching with his silent presence. Unfortunately, none of his disciples found freedom, but they founded 32 Buddhist schools.

People are clinging to teachers because they believe teachers could help them to freedom. There is nothing to teach about the inner world. As Bodhidharma once said, Freedom is "no knowledge."

There is nothing to heal or improve in the inner world; it is already perfect. However, its ideal state is covered with much trash. Teachers cannot help remove this trash because they and their teachings are trash and methods, seminars, and books. Only when you realize it, drop it all, and become your best and only teacher will you see the light of the Truth.

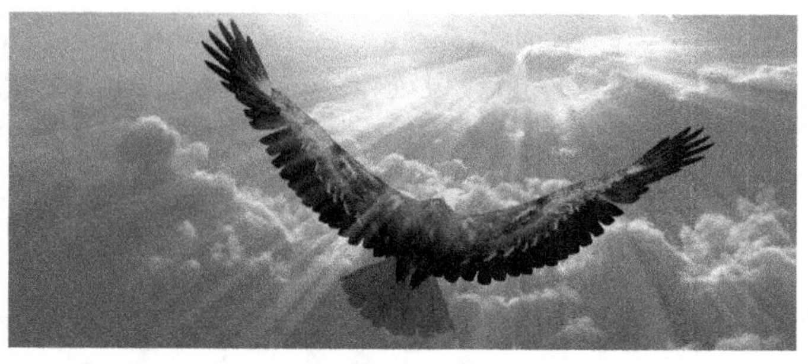

Knowing people is wisdom,
Knowing the Self is Enlightenment.
Mastering people requires force,
Mastering the Self needs strength

Tao Te Ching

Energy
Life is all about energy

If you want to find the secrets, think (in terms of) energy, frequency, and vibration.
Nikola Tesla

This chapter may seem confusing at first, but please bear with it. Read it through one more time; it will make sense eventually. It helps to think in terms of simple arithmetic.

An Intel-Star is a unique module that the writers of the Bible call the soul. It is attached to us <u>at the time of birth</u>. It departs at the time of death, loaded with our life experiences. See chapter *The Flower that Once has Blown.*

Intel-Star's outer Energoinformational field has an upper-frequency limit of 10 to the 67 power at 200% energy. It is the frequency and energy of the Enlightenment. Its lower limit is "0," or a point of death. An Intel-Star's energy level could drop as low as 4% (Adolf Hitler), corresponding to 10 to the 6 power frequency, characterizing human behavior.

With some exceptions, the frequency of the world and the Universe is 10 to the 56% Power (energy 100%), which is the frequency and energy level of what we call true Love. It is also the standard against which Intel-Star's percentage or energy level is calculated.

Science is not yet capable of registering true Love energy and frequency. It cannot locate Intel-Star. We can do it with *The Code of Life* and learn that Intel-Star's outer field frequency and corresponding energy level fluctuate, reflecting human behavior and mode of life.

Something in the Intel-Star never changes its core, which has 500% energy and 10 to the ten million Power frequency making Intel-Star indestructible. Intel-Star is "hanging" about one-half of one meter above our head. It keeps a record of our every experience in its outer field.

A newborn has Intel-Star's frequency and an energy level of true Love, potentially increasing it to 200% and 10 to the 67 Power frequency of Enlightenment. When brought up with Love, a child can exercise this potential and become their best teacher and doctor. It also means everyone has an equal opportunity to create a life of Health, Happiness, and Success regardless of the inheritance.

The nature of the Intel-Star energy and frequency is the same as in electricity. This energy has a greater frequency and a much higher upper limit than electricity. A person's Intel-Star energy level is the only accurate indicator of the person's goodness and vice. With *The SP (Star Pendulum)*, we determine it in just a few seconds, and later we do it without *The Code.*

The mechanics are quite simple. In the outer field of the Intel-Star, an energy level indicates our energoinformational state and what we are. It is not used for healing or any other purpose. A thermometer is a good example, as its mercury shows the number of degrees while the total amount of mercury remains the same at any degree. It is the same with the outer field of Intel-Star.

To avoid confusion, an outer field of the Intel-Star energy has nothing to do with the energy of the core of the Intel-Star. The energy of the outer field remains in the outer field of the Intel-Star. It demonstrates an individual level of goodness and vice and every character's quality. It does not show our physical energy.

Why is it so important to have a higher Intel-Star energy level? There are several reasons. The first is that the higher our energy level, the better humans we are. Another reason is that we will make fewer or no mistakes. Yet another reason is that we sooner get better answers related to every aspect of our life, including the right information on how to heal our body and brain ☺. The higher our Intel-Star energy level, the more powerful *Code* we are offered, which also means a more effective healing process.

<u>Depending on the nature of the question</u>, when using *The Code of Life,* we receive a reply demonstrating the person's level of personal qualities, including virtues, abilities, etc. For example:

- What is AB's level of physical energy at the moment? Reply 97%.

- How greedy is AB on a scale of 0 to 100%? Reply 3%.
- How loving is AB on a scale of 0 to 100%? Reply: 99%
- What is my life resource as of now? Reply 42 years.

It is necessary to use the Star Pendulum or Simplicity method to receive a reply.

Energy is waves of various lengths and frequencies. Love is a form of energy. Even the most solid objects are energy that vibrates with different frequencies, which can be measured. People's emotions and character qualities can be accurately measured only with the levels of Intel-Star energy.

The more intense is frequency, the more benevolent and constructive the corresponding energy. The intelligent energy of an unimaginable high frequency "created" our Universe. The intensity of the frequency of the Infinite Intelligence is impossible to determine with our means. What is amazing, it does not have a low limit. What is it that exists below zero frequency? It sounds like a Black Hole in the Universe.

Cancer cells have a 6% energy level, with a frequency of 10 to the 16 power. Coronavirus has 4% energy with a corresponding frequency of 10 to the 8 power—the lower the frequency, the longer and more destructive its energy waves. The higher the frequency, the higher the energy level, and the more benevolent, constructive, and healing. It is unimaginable goodness that must exist within Infinite Intelligence.

People have low Intel-Star energy levels mainly because they were not raised in a loving environment.

Inappropriate behavior and violation of the laws of nature lower the energy level. When the energy level is lower, its waves are longer and more destructive. They may disorient genes in several brain glands, prompting inappropriate behavior. Depending on their low energy levels, people would commit offenses, crimes, hut others, and, adhere to abnormal ways of living. Some people would do it unintentionally. People like Hitler, Obama, and Bush have been doing it purposefully. Whether intentionally or not, people do it because of their deficient energy level, with corresponding low IQ. In this book, we also explain how to raise the energy level.

Frequency is how often an event repeats itself over a set amount of time. In physics, the frequency of a wave is the number of wave crests that pass a point in one second (A wave crest is the wave's peak). Hertz (symbol Hz) is the unit measuring frequency. The higher the frequency, the shorter the wavelength. Short wavelengths are more energetic and have a higher penetrating power. They are also "manageable," meaning they can be focused. We use these higher frequencies with *The Code of Life* to focus its energy on pathogens and destroy them. In the Healing mode, we focus *The Code*'s energy on the causes of illness and destroy them.

Frequency makes energy benevolent or damaging. The lower the frequency, the more damaging it is to one's body, brain, and others. The lower the frequency (and corresponding energy), the longer its wave is. The longer the surge, the sooner its busting power damages the body and organs.

Low energy (below 52% and lower) is harmful and destructive. This harmful quality cannot be noticed at a 51%

level but gradually increases as energy and frequency drop. Energy above 52% is benevolent and constructive. Higher frequency/energy heals. People know little to nothing about the negative impact of low-frequency energy. Yet, they intuitively feel danger; It is the main reason why people who adhere to the laws of nature dislike and shy away from people who violate the laws of nature. People also know that Love heals.

The deficiency of energy is in itself a disease. At 4% of the energy level, one could be alive but very ill with cancer or a similar illness. Energy deficiency creates a fungus-like situation that allows pathogens to spread and consume the person.

Another issue is that one with less than 52% energy level would instinctively try to raise their energy level to be as far away as possible from "0" or the point of death by involuntarily sucking energy from other people. See *Energy Theft* in *Key points*. It is another reason why people who live by the laws of nature dislike and shy away from those who violate the laws of nature.

The lower one's energy level, the more unnatural the person is. People with deficient energy levels instinctively try to hide their despair under the pretense of happiness. They may appear friendly and agreeable but explode with anger and attack when something goes wrong. So how could one recognize a person with a low energy level?

One way to detect energy deficiency is to tell someone about *The Code of Life*. People with energy levels of 48% or less will reject it. They are afraid of Love and Truth that would expose their unfortunate state. Ask *The Code* how trustworthy people are when their energy level is below 15%. The best way to learn anything about a person in question without using the tools is to become a Master of Simplicity.

There is a separate issue. We cannot blame a snake for being a snake or a dog for being a dog. Likewise, we cannot blame people with deficient energy levels for being what they are. These people, more often than not, are powerless against their low energy. Negativity drives them despite their wish to change. Many testimonials on the Internet by low-energy people explain how plugged they are by psychological disorders.

Games of Thrones, *The Dutchman*, *Cats*, *Godfather*, thrillers, horror pictures, and similar "entertainment" are harmful, as they bombard the viewers with their creators' long waves/low-frequency energy. Low-energy humans create this "entertainment."

People with low energy know no love or happiness. They are invading countries, taking bribes, and endorsing pornography. They are creating nothing beneficial but destroying positive creation.

People with a high energy level made *Cinderella*, *Santa Claus*, *Moana*, *Puss in Boots*, *Apprentice*, Sandcastle, seven letters, *Le Petit Prince, and Avatar*. Unfortunately, only some good films were made amidst the sea of talented garbage.

I have known Vince since the time I lived in Toronto, Canada. He was a successful businessman. I did not see him for many years. Then, suddenly, I received a call from a mutual friend; she said Vince had hit rock bottom. He lived in a basement and did not talk to anyone; his relationship deteriorated with his wife and son.

My friend knew about me practicing *The Code of Life,* she told Vince about it, and Vince asked if I would help. Of course, I said, but remembering my lesson with Petro (see later in the book), I consulted *The Code of Life.* Today, I often know the reason before asking for *The Code.* Most of the time, it has been low energy. Again, my feeling was correct. Vince was doing something harmful. I didn't need to know the nature of the activity. It was essential to know that his energy level was 10%. I was not allowed to talk to him but could send an e-mail, which I did.

I wrote Vince that I could not help or even talk to him because he was involved in some unnatural harmful activity that he must quit damaging behavior for me to help. I have yet to hear from him again. Unfortunately it happens often when people with deficient energy levels refuse help by refusing to abandon their unnatural activity.

Various applications of *the Code* are explained throughout the book. Please read the entire book to understand how *The Code* performs, why and how you must charge it, the reason for the poem's recital, and other issues. You are charging not the request but *The Code.* Your charge will make it much more powerful, thus destroying anything that needs to be eliminated (pathogens, chemicals, wrong hormones, deposits of salts, Fat, Calcium, Cholesterol, and heavy metals). It will restore all that needs to be restored: organs, tissues, processes, systems, blood vessels, nerves, bones, and relationships.
The Code will dissolve stones and deposits, repair and reorient genes, and provide countless unique services. You

charge *The Code* with your energy by repeating for 30 seconds with emotion: *Thank you! Thank you! Thank you! Thank you!*

When filing a request, it is paramount to do it with a strong feeling: for the biocomputer to fulfill it.

When our energy level is between 52% and 80%, it is not powerful enough to destroy what needs to be destroyed and to restore what needs to be restored. So, we use *The Code's* energy to increase the power. When our energy is 80% and higher, we no longer charge *The Code* because our energy is sufficient to do the job.

The Code can only be used when your energy level is 52% (40% in some exceptional circumstances): "Raise your energy level," says Nature, "And you may enjoy my gifts."

However, a true gift is our inherent ability to heal without doctors and medications and raise our Intel-Star energy level without teachers and teachings. We do it when our energy is 80% and higher.

A request is necessary to program our Biocomputer with a task formulated in the request. In addition to our energy, our Biocomputer will focus *The Code's* energy on the target and accomplish the task. You charge *The Code* when it is so advised. When our energy is above 80%, our Biocomputer will complete the task without *The Code*.

Eventually, when our energy level is above 175%, we understand that The Codes were stepping stones to the realization that we have an inherent capability to diagnose, heal, and have the answer to any question without tools.

Inner Health is as important as physical health, for our physical health is only good when the Intel-Star energy level is high. We may feel great at lower energy levels, but this is misleading because when our energy level is lower than 80%, it could indicate some Health issues.

The Shield of Love. In the beginning, you can protect yourself from the low destructive energy of other people, negatively charged objects, and circumstances. Create a Shield of Love. To do so, you need to charge *The Code* when your energy is below 80%. Having your Intel-Star energy level above 80%, you would no longer need soap to wash your hands and body; it would be enough to rinse it with water. As to your hair, use only baking soda. Every shampoo, soap, cream, etc., contain harmful chemicals, toothpaste, and dental rinse, except floss.

Being in the state of Love, Oh Love, I request your infinite power to restore my energy system and create the Shield of Love to protect me from negative influence.

Create the shield once and activate it when necessary:

Being in the state of Love, Oh Love, I request thy infinite power to activate my Shield of Love.

Life is simple when we do not complicate it with our limited minds clogged by religion, teachers, and teachings. So, discard all teachers and teaching, make the mind stark naked, and enjoy the simplicity of life you were born to experience.

As the Beatles say in their world's famous song, All You Need is Love: Easy…All You Need is Love. Love is all you need.

To be protected by the shield, your energy level must be 52% and higher.

<u>Example of energy levels and related IQ:</u>

Roosevelt **86; 136 IQ**
James Madison, Father of the US Constitution **89; 138 IQ**
George Washington **86; 132 IQ**
The 55 Delegates to the United States
Constitutional Convention **77**
1797, George Washington government **61**
Adams **57**
La Sisi **56; 122 IQ**
Donald Trump **58; 125 IQ**
Maduro **56% 121 IQ**
Xi Jinping **56% 128 IQ**
British Royal family, including Diana, **7%**

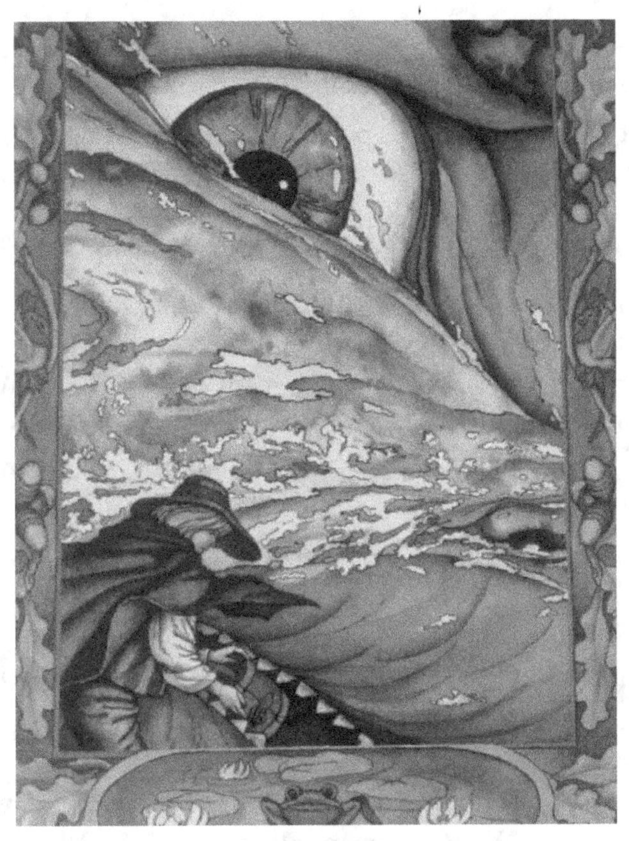

The gift
By Anna and Nadia Balzhak

The Code of Life
The Intel-Star (soul) energy level is the only accurate
indicator of the person's goodness and vice.

The Code is at the core of our Biocomputer and Life. It was
waiting to be discovered. It is active during our life regardless
of our knowledge of it. When used consciously, *The Code of
Life* becomes our guiding star leading us to ever-higher

25

energy levels to become self-contained, self-sufficient human beings.

Most information in the book is written for people with 52% - - 79% energy levels, as most people fall within these energy levels. The book also explains how to raise your energy and greatly benefit yourself.

When your energy level is 100%, *The Code of Life* will enable you to utilize fifty percent of the Biocomputer's capability instead of an average of five percent. When our energy level is 198%, we use 80 percent of the Biocomputer's power. It empowers you with control of your Health, relationships, business, and finances – your life of happiness.

The higher your energy level and corresponding frequency, the more benevolent its power is. As explained later, a human with an 80% energy level no longer identifies contaminants but destroys causes. There is no need to place their hands on *The Code* in the morning and before bed.

You may start your day with this request (edit the request as appropriate). When the energy level is below80%:

Being in the state of Love, Oh Love, I request thy infinite power to charge my Code of Life with the full strength of thy energy to provide me with the means to create a life of Health, Happiness, and Success. Thank you! Thank you! Thank you! Keep charging *The Code* for 30 seconds.

When your energy is 80%:
Being in the state of Love, Oh Love, I request thy infinite power to provide me with the means to create a life of Health, Happiness, and Success.

Always **ask** *The Code* if you could charge it with a particular request and what kind of energy to use (the energy of Love or Infinite Intelligence.)

The Code advised sending the President this letter in the third month of the pandemic. *"I am an American writer and researcher living in Hurghada, Egypt. We developed a system, The Code of Life Communications and System of Health, to speed up the US economic recovery time five times. Sixty-eight percent of Americans, including children and seniors, are immune from COVID-19. No masks, sprays, or other precautions are necessary for these people. They cannot transfer the virus.*
Sixty-five percent of American working adults are immune to COVID-19."

It could be a coincidence, but soon, President Trump decided to open the US economy.

Like fish in the sea, we live in the ocean of Infinite Intelligence, which is also the Field of Infinite Knowledge. We need to become conscious of this state, which happens when we are peaceful with high energy levels. To have the energy level we call True Love (and higher) is the only condition necessary to build a truly happy life. No method will ever help your happiness and Freedom unless it enables you to increase your energy level beyond 100%.

Everything in Nature has a True Love's energy level vibrating with ten to the 56 power frequency. When a baby is born, it has a 100% energy level vibrating with 10 to the 56 power. When it is baptized, its energy drops to 60%. It drops because the baby was initiated into something that is not true. Nature does not compromise. Unfortunately, from day one, Love in many people begins to sink into the sea of ignorance.

According to 2017 US statistics, 75% of American children are brought up in an environment devoid of love, which is parental ignorance bordering on stupidity because lack of love in childhood drastically reduces the opportunity for a child to create a life of happiness in the future.

The Code of Life utilizes energy with the frequency of 10^{56} Hz. The frequency of the state of Freedom is 10^{67} Hz. Science cannot register such frequencies, but a Master of Simplicity and the SP can. It vibrates with higher frequencies than the body's emotions thoughts and pathogens/parasites. Cancer, for example, has a low frequency of 10^{16} Intense hate is at 10^{17}. It is incredible how the two (cancer and hate), seemingly unrelated, vibrate with almost the same frequency. Does it not tell us something? The saber-waver John McCain spent most of his life intensely hating enemies; he died of a brain tumor.

I keep exploring *The Code of Life* – a goldmine of the right knowledge. Like all life and the Universe, *The Code* has 100% energy in its free state. To heal ourselves, we are charging *The Code* with additional energy. Something inexplicable happens as our charge of *The Code of Life* multiplies its initial charge many a hundred times. It is a mystery how a bunch of zeros arranged in a particular manner and printed on paper generate such high-frequency energy.

Here is an example of how *The Code* is fulfilling our request. We program our Biocomputer (brain) with the request to destroy worms in the digestive system:

Being in the state of Love, Oh Love, I request thy infinite power to charge my Code of Life with the full strength of thy energy to destroy worms in my digestive system and restore it to perfection of health.

We charge *The Code* for 30 seconds, saying with emotion: Thank you! Thank you! Thank you!

With this request, our Biocomputer focuses the energy of *The Code* (in addition to our energy) on a given task: the destruction of the worms.

How *The Code* is accomplishing this phenomenal task is a puzzle. Try to solve it☺

Being the Master of Simplicity or using the SP, you would check whether *The Code* is charged 100% or needs an additional charge. Thirty seconds of the intense charge will guarantee 100%. The Code will not be fully active when charged less than 100%. You could also verify whether any pathogens remain in your digestive tract.

Depending on your energy level, it may take just one request or several days of repeating it four times a day to get rid of pathogens. The higher your energy level, the less time you need to eliminate pathogens.

Later I learned *The Code* stays charged and keeps silently "working" for eighteen hours. It works with its high-frequency energy of 10 to the 6000 power.
The number of charges per day and number of days is usually less than it was initially calculated:

- When as in the above example, *The Code* would complete the process earlier than it was programmed.
- When *The Code* wants us to relax to receive a vital message.
- When we make a mistake in determining the number of days.

It happened to me several times when I was initially told to charge *The Code*, for example, for five days, and suddenly, when the symptoms were still present, I was asked to stop charging *The Code*. In every case, the symptoms were still there. I obeyed the command and stopped charging. In a few days, the symptoms were gone without charge. It is inexplicable why and how it happens; luckily, I always discover something new about *The Code of Life*. That is why it is vital to become a Master of Simplicity or master the SP to monitor the process. It is all a fun thing to do. My nine-year-old granddaughter Eren learned the SP in one day.

The Code can be used to heal without the SP or be the Master of Simplicity when you know what to heal.

Anything you wish to accomplish may be accurately checked with the *Simplicity Method,* or the SP, initially held over *The Code of Life* to ensure the reply's accuracy. *For example,* "Do I need to brush my teeth with toothpaste?" NO (by the way, it is never "yes" for toothpaste). "With H2O2?" NO. "With toothpowder?" NO.

The Code of Life confirms that if you want to save your teeth, throw out all dental tools, including toothpaste, brushes, rinsing, etc. Sparingly use only floss. Do not rinse your mouth. A mouth has a perfect environment that 100%

protects teeth from bacteria. Every piece of dental paraphernalia destroys this ideal environment. If you have some tooth discomfort, it is bacteria or protozoa. Instantly destroy it with *The Code*. Honey and dark chocolate are good for the teeth, as the mouth's environment is sweet. It is not sweets that create problems for your teeth but dental garbage. You will have no odor as the environment eliminates it. Some film (thin coating) may cover teeth. It is your protection from bacteria that is destroyed by toothpaste.

Dentures should be brushed with and kept overnight in warm water. Do not use a denture cleanser (it is a poison), only a hard brush! Confirm it all with The Code. I have practiced it for a long time.

You will see a dentist never again. However, because there was much damage done to teeth during a lifetime, you may need to have a denture, partial, or a crown. Be very careful with using a crown. Do not listen to a dentist. They are guessing, and too many have a low Intel-Star energy level, which means poor diagnosis. Consult your *Code* on where you need a crown. But, above all, choose a dentist with a high energy level when it comes to crowns. Veneers destroy teeth. Implants are very bad for your health; they totally destroy the mouth's natural environment. Listen to your *Code*, not a dentist.

Do not try to consult a dentist on this issue. Always consult The Code. In the US, many dentists are paid by toothpaste producers to promote this damaging garbage. It destroys teeth like <u>every</u> shampoo will make you eventually lose hair. Wash your hair only with baking soda. It is safe.

With the SP or Simplicity method, you can accurately determine the necessity and the amount of salt, sugar, pepper, and spices your body (not your mind☺) needs. In addition, you will know if a person is worthy of the relationship.

"Do I need to file a request to clean up my pharynx from pathogens?" "Yes." "How many times?" "Three times." That is when your energy is 52% to 80%. When it is above 80%: Use the energy of Love to destroy all causes inhibiting the pharynx and restore its health. The nose stops running as soon as you file the first request.

"Did Jenifer go to Sacramento on business?" No.

In the past, I used canned tuna for salads. Just a few days ago, I made tuna salad. After I made it, I tested it for contaminants. To my surprise, there were pathogens in the salad. The tuna was not just bad; it was very bad. It has never happened before with canned tuna in water. I had to throw the salad. This example should tell you to be careful and test every ingredient you use. It is specially important thing to do by seniours. Salt, sugar, and spices could be contaminated. Clean them by placing them on top of *The Code of Horus*. You also may use it in the fridge and counters regardless of your Intel-Star energy level.

"Did Oswald kill President Kennedy?" YES. "Where the Republicans behind this murder?" NO. "Was the KGB behind this murder?" NO. "Where Democrats behind this murder?" YES. "Where Democrats behind Robert Kennedy murder?" YES. Thus, you can unveil any mystery. We cannot have conventional proof of many things we discover, but some discoveries may lead to investigation and be proven this way.

I would not encourage you to ask this question because it wastes time. The only reason I did it was because many years ago, while making *Inside the KGB* special for

NBC television network, I interviewed Semichastny, the director of the KGB, at the time when Kennedy was murdered.

The question was sensitive because Oswald, who shot Kennedy, spent much time in the USSR and married a Russian girl. Leisurely, Semichastny was telling me Oswald was a lousy shot and would never be able to kill anything at such a distance. I was suspicious but had no means to verify it. When I later checked it with *The Code of Life,* the answers were, "Oswald was a perfect shot. He killed Kennedy. Semichastny was lying." No wonder, Semichastny's energy level was 12%.

I never trusted Soviet information about Hitler's death. *The Code* confirmed Hitler, Eva, and a few other fascists escaped Germany on a submarine and landed in Chile, where a house was waiting for them in a secluded area. The house is still there, along with a sub guarded by the Chilean government. It would become a tourist attraction with time, poisoning people with its long destructive waves.

Hitler died of cancer when he was 67. It is another puzzle, an exception. How did this man live that long with a 4% energy level and cancer? Hitler's issue proves there is always room for exceptions. Eva Braun, Hitler's wife, lived until she was 81. Today, only one alive person is there, a 101-year-old crew member. It brings to mind another exclusion: John D. Rockefeller, a greedy person with a 14% energy level, was determined to live 100 years despite being ill during his first fifty years.

Rockefeller's energy level has been increasing since he was 80 years old. He was doing something for his inner growth.

However, it would take much time to determine what he was doing.

It was 74% at the time of Rockefeller's death. He died when he was 99.

While healing can be accomplished without mastering simplicity or the SP, it must be used to diagnose, receive feedback, test, etc., or receive answers to queries.

Here is your request for a long life. Translate it into English and adjust accordingly

Блажен кто жизни-любви чашу полную допьет до дна как тот бокал вина,

И кто роман её волшебный дочтет до самого конца!

(your name) допьёт, (your name) дочтёт, (your name) здоровой проживет.

Ещё счастливых много лет, до ста семнадцати годов (set the years) заветного конца.

Say it every morning upon waking.

The Code of Life ™

```
000000000  000000000  000000000  000000000  000000000  000000000  000000000  000000000  000000000  000000000
000000000  000000000  000000000  000000000  000000000  000000000  000000000  000000000  000000000  000000000
000000000  000000000  000000000  000000000  000000000  000000000  000000000  000000000  000000000  000000000
000000000  000000000  000000000  000000000  000000000  000000000  000000000  000000000  000000000  000000000
000000000  000000000  000000000  000000000  000000000  000000000  000000000  000000000  000000000  000000000
000000000  000000000  000000000  000000000  000000000  000000000  000000000  000000000  000000000  000000000
000000000  000000000  000000000  000000000  000000000  000000000  000000000  000000000  000000000  000000000
000000000  000000000  000000000  000000000  000000000  000000000  000000000  000000000  000000000  000000000
000000000  000000000  000000000  000000000  000000000  000000000  000000000  000000000  000000000  000000000
000000000  000000000  000000000  000000000  000000000  000000000  000000000  000000000  000000000  000000000
000000000  000000000  000000000  000000000  000000000  000000000  000000000  000000000  000000000  000000000
000000000  000000000  000000000  000000000  000000000  000000000  000000000  000000000  000000000  000000000
000000000  000000000  000000000  000000000  000000000  000000000  000000000  000000000  000000000  000000000
000000000  000000000  000000000  000000000  000000000  000000000  000000000  000000000  000000000  000000000
000000000  000000000  000000000  000000000  000000000  000000000  000000000  000000000  000000000  000000000
000000000  000000000  000000000  000000000  000000000  000000000  000000000  000000000  000000000  000000000
000000000  000000000  000000000  000000000  000000000  000000000  000000000  000000000  000000000  000000000
000000000  000000000  000000000  000000000  000000000  000000000  000000000  000000000  000000000  000000000

000000000  000000000  000000000  000000000  000000000  000000000  000000000  000000000  000000000  000000000
000000000  000000000  000000000  000000000  000000000  000000000  000000000  000000000  000000000  000000000
```

```
000000000  000000000  000000000  000000000  000000000  000000000  000000000  000000000  000000000  000000000
000000000  000000000  000000000  000000000  000000000  000000000  000000000  000000000  000000000  000000000
000000000  000000000  000000000  000000000  000000000  000000000  000000000  000000000  000000000  000000000
000000000  000000000  000000000  000000000  000000000  000000000  000000000  000000000  000000000  000000000
000000000  000000000  000000000  000000000  000000000  000000000  000000000  000000000  000000000  000000000
000000000  000000000  000000000  000000000  000000000  000000000  000000000  000000000  000000000  000000000
000000000  000000000  000000000  000000000  000000000  000000000  000000000  000000000  000000000  000000000
000000000  000000000  000000000  000000000  000000000  000000000  000000000  000000000  000000000  000000000
000000000  000000000  000000000  000000000  000000000  000000000  000000000  000000000  000000000  000000000
000000000  000000000  000000000  000000000  000000000  000000000  000000000  000000000  000000000  000000000
000000000  000000000  000000000  000000000  000000000  000000000  000000000  000000000  000000000  000000000
000000000  000000000  000000000  000000000  000000000  000000000  000000000  000000000  000000000  000000000
000000000  000000000  000000000  000000000  000000000  000000000  000000000  000000000  000000000  000000000
000000000  000000000  000000000  000000000  000000000  000000000  000000000  000000000  000000000  000000000
000000000  000000000  000000000  000000000  000000000  000000000  000000000  000000000  000000000  000000000
000000000  000000000  000000000  000000000  000000000  000000000  000000000  000000000  000000000  000000000
000000000  000000000  000000000  000000000  000000000  000000000  000000000  000000000  000000000  000000000

000000000  000000000  000000000  000000000  000000000  000000000  000000000  000000000  000000000  000000000
000000000  000000000  000000000  000000000  000000000  000000000  000000000  000000000  000000000  000000000
000000000  000000000  000000000  000000000  000000000  000000000  000000000  000000000  000000000  000000000
000000000  000000000  000000000  000000000  000000000  000000000  000000000  000000000  000000000  000000000
000000000  000000000  000000000  000000000  000000000  000000000  000000000  000000000  000000000  000000000
000000000  000000000  000000000  000000000  000000000  000000000  000000000  000000000  000000000  000000000
000000000  000000000  000000000  000000000  000000000  000000000  000000000  000000000  000000000  000000000
000000000  000000000  000000000  000000000  000000000  000000000  000000000  000000000  000000000  000000000
000000000  000000000  000000000  000000000  000000000  000000000  000000000  000000000  000000000  000000000
000000000  000000000  000000000  000000000  000000000  000000000  000000000  000000000  000000000  000000000
000000000  000000000  000000000  000000000  000000000  000000000  000000000  000000000  000000000  000000000
000000000  000000000  000000000  000000000  000000000  000000000  000000000  000000000  000000000  000000000
000000000  000000000  000000000  000000000  000000000  000000000  000000000  000000000  000000000  000000000
000000000  000000000  000000000  000000000  000000000  000000000  000000000  000000000  000000000  000000000
000000000  000000000  000000000  000000000  000000000  000000000  000000000  000000000  000000000  000000000
000000000  000000000  000000000  000000000  000000000  000000000  000000000  000000000  000000000  000000000
000000000  000000000  000000000  000000000  000000000  000000000  000000000  000000000  000000000  000000000
000000000  000000000  000000000  000000000  000000000  000000000  000000000  000000000  000000000  000000000
000000000  000000000  000000000  000000000  000000000  000000000  000000000  000000000  000000000  000000000
000000000  000000000  000000000  000000000  000000000  000000000  000000000  000000000  000000000  000000000

000000000  000000000  000000000  000000000  000000000  000000000  000000000  000000000  000000000  000000000
000000000  000000000  000000000  000000000  000000000  000000000  000000000  000000000  000000000  000000000
000000000  000000000  000000000  000000000  000000000  000000000  000000000  000000000  000000000  000000000
000000000  000000000  000000000  000000000  000000000  000000000  000000000  000000000  000000000  000000000
000000000  000000000  000000000  000000000  000000000  000000000  000000000  000000000  000000000  000000000
000000000  000000000  000000000  000000000  000000000  000000000  000000000  000000000  000000000  000000000
000000000  000000000  000000000  000000000  000000000  000000000  000000000  000000000  000000000  000000000
000000000  000000000  000000000  000000000  000000000  000000000  000000000  000000000  000000000  000000000
000000000  000000000  000000000  000000000  000000000  000000000  000000000  000000000  000000000  000000000
000000000  000000000  000000000  000000000  000000000  000000000  000000000  000000000  000000000  000000000
000000000  000000000  000000000  000000000  000000000  000000000  000000000  000000000  000000000  000000000
000000000  000000000  000000000  000000000  000000000  000000000  000000000  000000000  000000000  000000000
000000000  000000000  000000000  000000000  000000000  000000000  000000000  000000000  000000000  000000000
000000000  000000000  000000000  000000000  000000000  000000000  000000000  000000000  000000000  000000000
000000000  000000000  000000000  000000000  000000000  000000000  000000000  000000000  000000000  000000000
000000000  000000000  000000000  000000000  000000000  000000000  000000000  000000000  000000000  000000000
000000000  000000000  000000000  000000000  000000000  000000000  000000000  000000000  000000000  000000000
000000000  000000000  000000000  000000000  000000000  000000000  000000000  000000000  000000000  000000000

000000000  000000000  000000000  000000000  000000000  000000000  000000000  000000000  000000000  000000000
000000000  000000000  000000000  000000000  000000000  000000000  000000000  000000000  000000000  000000000
000000000  000000000  000000000  000000000  000000000  000000000  000000000  000000000  000000000  000000000
000000000  000000000  000000000  000000000  000000000  000000000  000000000  000000000  000000000  000000000
000000000  000000000  000000000  000000000  000000000  000000000  000000000  000000000  000000000  000000000
000000000  000000000  000000000  000000000  000000000  000000000  000000000  000000000  000000000  000000000
000000000  000000000  000000000  000000000  000000000  000000000  000000000  000000000  000000000  000000000
000000000  000000000  000000000  000000000  000000000  000000000  000000000  000000000  000000000  000000000
000000000  000000000  000000000  000000000  000000000  000000000  000000000  000000000  000000000  000000000
000000000  000000000  000000000  000000000  000000000  000000000  000000000  000000000  000000000  000000000
000000000  000000000  000000000  000000000  000000000  000000000  000000000  000000000  000000000  000000000
000000000  000000000  000000000  000000000  000000000  000000000  000000000  000000000  000000000  000000000
000000000  000000000  000000000  000000000  000000000  000000000  000000000  000000000  000000000  000000000
000000000  000000000  000000000  000000000  000000000  000000000  000000000  000000000  000000000  000000000
000000000  000000000  000000000  000000000  000000000  000000000  000000000  000000000  000000000  000000000
000000000  000000000  000000000  000000000  000000000  000000000  000000000  000000000  000000000  000000000
000000000  000000000  000000000  000000000  000000000  000000000  000000000  000000000  000000000  000000000
000000000  000000000  000000000  000000000  000000000  000000000  000000000  000000000  000000000  000000000

000000000  000000000  000000000  000000000  000000000  000000000  000000000  000000000  000000000  000000000
000000000  000000000  000000000  000000000  000000000  000000000  000000000  000000000  000000000  000000000
000000000  000000000  000000000  000000000  000000000  000000000  000000000  000000000  000000000  000000000
000000000  000000000  000000000  000000000  000000000  000000000  000000000  000000000  000000000  000000000
000000000  000000000  000000000  000000000  000000000  000000000  000000000  000000000  000000000  000000000
000000000  000000000  000000000  000000000  000000000  000000000  000000000  000000000  000000000  000000000
000000000  000000000  000000000  000000000  000000000  000000000  000000000  000000000  000000000  000000000
```

```
000000000   000000000   000000000   000000000   000000000   000000000   000000000   000000000   000000000   000000000
000000000   000000000   000000000   000000000   000000000   000000000   000000000   000000000   000000000   000000000
000000000   000000000   000000000   000000000   000000000   000000000   000000000   000000000   000000000   000000000
000000000   000000000   000000000   000000000   000000000   000000000   000000000   000000000   000000000   000000000
000000000   000000000   000000000   000000000   000000000   000000000   000000000   000000000   000000000   000000000
000000000   000000000   000000000   000000000   000000000   000000000   000000000   000000000   000000000   000000000
000000000   000000000   000000000   000000000   000000000   000000000   000000000   000000000   000000000   000000000
000000000   000000000   000000000   000000000   000000000   000000000   000000000   000000000   000000000   000000000
000000000   000000000   000000000   000000000   000000000   000000000   000000000   000000000   000000000   000000000
000000000   000000000   000000000   000000000   000000000   000000000   000000000   000000000   000000000   000000000
000000000   000000000   000000000   000000000   000000000   000000000   000000000   000000000   000000000   000000000
```

X 50000000000000000000000000000000000000

The Code of Life may get distorted in Kindle. Here is what it should be:

The Code consists of ten columns. Each column is made of six primary codes. Each primary Code is made of 18 rows, nine zeros each. At the bottom of *the Code*, there is a row of digits:

X 50000000000000000000000000000000000000

The Code of Life has been available to humanity forever. I discovered it; I did not create it. I named it *The Code of Life* because, in its free state, the *Code's* frequency is the frequency of Nature, the Universe, and true Love. It is given to us to live by the energy of Love, enjoy Love's benefits, and battle negativity. In reality, there is no need to battle negativity; all we need to do is raise our energy level. The higher it is, the sooner negativity evaporates.

To use *The Code of Life,* you need to print it on both sides of one page.

When your energy level is above 80%, use the one page of *The Code of Horus* printed on both sides of the page. However, you do not charge The Code with this energy but destroy "all causes inhibiting my lever," as an example.

No one with an energy level below 52% can use *The Code* (some exceptions apply.) It is another lock created by evolution to encourage people to increase their energy levels.

Recently I discovered even more powerful codes, including *The Code of Horus+*, described in the chapter *Fountain of Youth: The Code of Horus and The Tree of Life.* I used it for a while and then was advised to abandon it.

With *The Code of Life,* you enter a dimension where you can know all truths. It is the world of higher energy, true knowledge, and happiness. Some of life's disappointments may still happen, yet, even disappointments will be to your advantage, if not instantly.

No distance exists in the state of Oneness: everything is instantly here and now, providing our Intel-Star energy level of 100%. Like Freedom, Oneness cannot be explained; it can only be experienced.

When your Intel-Star energy level is 100% and more, you can aid an ailing person even when this person is on the other side of the globe. It is possible because of Oneness.

1941 was the most challenging year for Russia, with fascists rats announcing they would defeat the USSR in a few days. Russia was never defeated. In WWII, Russia lost twenty million lives. Hence, the following poem by Simonov:

Wait for me, and I'll come back!
Wait with all you've got!
Wait, when dreary yellow rains
Tell you, you should not.
Wait, when snow is falling fast,

Wait, when summer's hot,
Wait, when yesterdays are past,
Others are forgotten.
Even when my dearest ones
Say that I am lost,
Even when my friends give up,
Sit and count the cost,
Drink a glass of bitter wine
To the fallen friend -
Wait! And do not drink with them!
Wait until the end!

Wait for me, and I'll come back,
Dodging every fate!
"What a bit of luck!" they'll say,
Those that would not wait.
They will never understand
How amidst the strife,
By your waiting for me, darling,
You had saved my life.
Only you and I will know
How you got me through.
Simply - you knew how to wait -
No one else but you.

These three lines exemplify Oneness:

How amidst the strife,
By your waiting for me, dear,
You had saved my life.

Is it possible to save by waiting for the soldier, fighting thousands of miles away from home? Oneness provides for this opportunity. It must be exceptional, extraordinary, and unwavering waiting to make it happen. For this phenomenon to happen, each person involved must have their Intel-Steal energy above 170%. You also may recite this poem when you are ill, believing "you" will come back to health

On one occasion, I was doing on-railing pushups on my deck in Egypt. Suddenly, I heard a loud chirping and saw a small bird of heavenly beauty sitting a few feet away, chirping. It was a parrot with feathers shining with every rainbow color. I introduced myself to the bird and got more chirping in reply. We talked like this for a few minutes, and then the parrot was gone – flew away and had never returned. There must be some good message there, a thought crossed my mind. Indeed, the next day I received news about a long-standing problem was resolved. It was Oneness that facilitated the information.

Someone wondered if *The Code* could be used with bad intentions. You could guess the reply. The one with bad intentions would have an energy level below 52%. *The Code* can be employed only with a 52% energy level and higher.

Place a jar of tap water on top of *The Code*. It would be made alive in ten to twenty minutes with a PH of around 7,2. *The Code* could purify water and do many other "miracles." These are not miracles but the law. Like many other "unusual" happenings, it is still beyond science. However, even *The Code* cannot make the LA tap water drinkable. It is overloaded with chemicals and cannot be purified with *The Code of Life* or *Horus*.

It is imperative to neutralize the subconscious negativity's influence, as is explained in the Key Points. It is a win-win situation because you will gain The Code's power and enjoy your life's journey.

Because the energy level is 300% in its free state, *The Code* keeps working even without being charged. When it is charged, its energy jumps to 700%. *The Code of Horus* will eliminate toxins and parasites when the foodstuff is placed on top or in the refrigerator.

You must check whether to use *The Code of Horus* or *The Code of Life*. Eventually, you will need no code.

Interestingly, *The Code of Life* or *Horus* will destroy all "bad" stuff while leaving intact nutrients, vitamins, and minerals, all that is good. How does it make the right choice, and what are mechanics of the process?

With *The Code of Life*, you could make another request or repeat the same request in two hours and thirty minutes unless directed otherwise. The pause's length also depends on individual qualities, the state of health, and the energy level. These factors can only be determined using the SP or Mastering Simplicity.

If you did not yet master it and are not a Master of Simplicity, charge your Code four times a day until you feel cured. These numbers also depend on your energy level.

The initial evolutionary design was created to safeguard humanity from destruction, enabling us to utilize higher energy to implement lasting change. True, a powerful human mind can foster change that is not beneficial. Such change would be relatively short-lived, as positive action would nullify the negative results. The positive evolution is forever, despite the temporary negative setbacks.

Human evolution also has another safety lock. When someone lives on low energy, it will result in stress. Stress causes invasion of pathogens that attack organs, virus disorients and damages genes, which would eventually cause a deadly illness.

The Universe, with all life, is immersed in the ocean of *Infinite Intelligence,* which religious people call God or Allah. Our Biocomputer is connected 24/7 to *Infinite Intelligence* via receptors in the brain. If our belief contradicts truthful information stored in the *Infinite Intelligence,* psychological conflict is created, resulting in tension, and stress. Depending on the intensity of the long wave's low-frequency energy, it could eventually damage the organs.

The Code is a powerful system. Always ask where you should place it, whether you need to have it in your bedroom, have it with you, or if you need to charge it with a particular request. Do not ever use *The Code* without asking it for permission.

Before I discovered *The Code of Horus,* I was advised to use my *Code of Life* only remotely at some point. I knew from experience that there would be a surprise or a discovery when some unusual advice dawned. Inevitably, a few days later, I was advised never to use *The Code* again and to destroy it along with all copies. After making some inquiries, I got the message: the inherent quality of knowing without tools and healing myself without doctors and medicine became active.

I placed several copies of my *Code* (one page only) in the refrigerator to ensure the foodstuff was constantly cleansed. *The Code* also eliminates odors in the fridge and freezer. I also put a copy of *The Code* on top of the counter and placed water, grains, fruits, and vegetables on top of it for about 15 minutes. Everything remained the same, except there was no longer a need to file requests or inquiries with the paper *Code*. Later, I was directed to use *The Code of Horus*, then The Star Code, then The Code Horus +, and, finally, not to use any *Code*. It all could be different for you; maybe you won't need any *Code* much sooner than I .

When I say "I was advised," it means that my request was approved. There are still many puzzles with *The Code*. We would guess them one after another and update the book with new information.

I suggest printing several copies of *The Code* and keeping them at all times - in the freezer and refrigerator, on a counter, and some kitchen shelves.

Once in Egypt, my refrigerator started leaking inside. We called for service. I put *The Code* in the fridge (and in the freezer) solely for cleaning food and killing odors. When the service person arrived, he did not find any leak. Since then, the refrigerator has been working fine.

When your confidence in *The Code* becomes unshakable; you will be guided in every step. Several conditions will apply depending on one's state of health, energy level, and experience.

- Your energy level must be not less than 150% to use your inherent ability to communicate and make inquiries without tools and heal yourself without doctors and medicines.
- *The Code* provided in the book must be used extensively for 12 months unless you are advised to use a more powerful *Code*.

- You must become proficient at healing with *The Code* alone and without using doctors, medicines, and equipment.
- You must use SP or Master the method of Simplicity.

Some stupid people believe *The Code* is Black Magic. Fortunately, Black magic's idea exists nowhere except in an ignorant mind, for the low energy people are incapable of magic. Anyone trying to hurt another person has a low energy level and cannot use *The Code*.

Restrictions

These are the essential things I learned through trial and error. I ask you not to make the same mistakes and pay close attention to the following:

1. Never try to learn anything about another human being without their permission. It includes information about the state of their health.

   a. You can obtain information about another person(s) when you know this person(s) is planning to hurt others.

   b. You may enquire about other people only in relation to yourself.

   c. You may obtain any information about public figures, including their sexual preference. Wikipedia describes a public figure as a person, such as a politician, celebrity, social media personality, or business leader, with a certain social position within a certain scope and a significant influence.

d. You can ask, "Did Obama receive bribes from Saudis for selling them arms?" You cannot ask if Hillary Clinton is a fraud. You may ask if Hillary is an honest person.

e. You also may ask if any historical personality, document, dogma, record, or scripture is accurate and of any dead person's energy level.

f. Always **ask** the SP if you could request the answer to the particular question.

2. You may not inquire about another person's personal qualities unless you have a business or some relationship with this person or this person is a public figure. You could make these inquiries about your relatives.

3. Do not try to heal anyone without their request/permission.

4. Do not make inquiries requested by someone regarding someone else.

5. We must have no emotions present while using *The Code*.

6. *The Code* can be used extensively for diagnoses and healing. It should be used sparingly for the "negative" inquiries about people with low energy levels and negative events like wars, riots, lootings, etc. When you still do it extensively, you may temporarily weaken the body and experience the lightness of the head.

When you violate the rules, you may err in your inquiries. You could disorient or even damage genes in the brain. I have no idea why it happens. I discovered it accidentally and had to spend some time restoring genes.

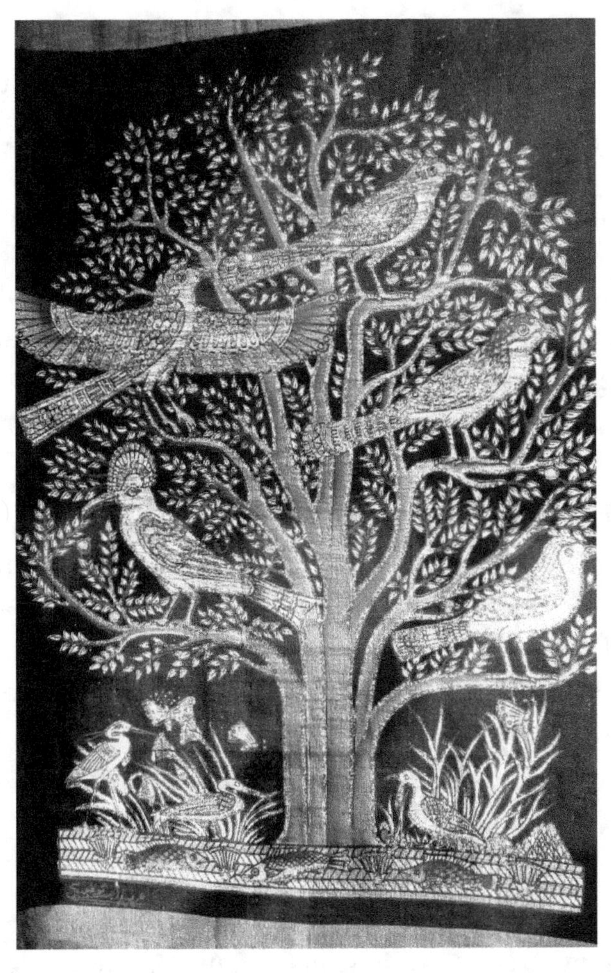

Fountain of Youth: The Code of Horus and the Tree of life System

The inspiring atmosphere of Egypt, created by friendly people, warm weather, and blue waters of the Red Sea, blended with the ever-moving fiery barchans of the Sahara Desert, was responsible for almost all my books. This time I came to Egypt to discover two great Egyptian treasures, The Code of Horus and the Tree of Life, which resulted in the discovery of *The Code of Horus and the Tree of life System: Fountain of Youth.*

Traveling in this unusual mysterious country, I took thousands of pictures of temples and the Sahara Desert. In December 2020, seemingly for no reason, I was browsing through my great collection and, ostensibly for no reason, singled out a picture of Horus and measured its energy. Amazingly, the image of Horus yielded a 300% energy level.

Only people with 150% Intel-Star energy level and higher could use *The Code of Horus and the Tree of life System*. It is another reminder aimed at the rest of humanity: raise your Intel-Star energy level, and you will find what you are looking for.

In ancient Egypt, Horus was a god in the form of a falcon whose right eye is the sun or morning star, representing power and an essence: Intel-Star (soul), whose left eye is the moon or evening star, representing healing.

Though alive, a tree or an animal does not have Intel-Star. They have only lower energy we call physical from food. Anything created by humans, a building, an image, or any object will have the energy of the creator(s), which means the creators of Horus' image were highly advanced human beings. Yet, there is another puzzle here. The maximum Intel-Star energy level a human could have is 200% -- a level of enlightenment. How then does the image of Horus have a 300% energy level?

As always, there are exceptions. For example, when an image (a picture or statue) of a real person is created by an artist who has a low Intel-Star energy level (Roerich (40%),

Rembrandt (37%), Van Gogh (6%), the created image would have an Intel-Star energy level of the portrayed person, and not of the artist. As a side issue, Roerich had many problems with his famous travel to Tibet. The actual reason was his low Intel-Star energy level. Tibetan monks (an overall 86% energy level) knew nothing about Intel-Star levels, but they sensed Roerich's low damaging energy and did not want him there.

According to *The Code,* Egyptian people did not know about Horus' energy and qualities. Still, priests knew something about it and used it to learn the truth about anyone, verify information from the past and present, and heal people.

As you already know, True Love and its 10 to the 56 Power frequency is our measurement system's standard and starting point. From this point down, when the frequency decreases, the energy decreases until it becomes Zero or a point of no existence. When the frequency increases, it makes the system more powerful. The higher the frequency, the greater the efficiency of healing and research. It does not have an upper limit. At least, I was not able to determine it.

How do we know true Love and its 10 to the 56 Power frequency is a true measurement system's standard? By using logic and common sense. For example, Hitler's energy level was 4%, Obama's 9%, Bush's 6%, Stalin's 5%, and Roosevelt's about 90%. You know what these people have done. The "energy level" measurement system is accurate, unlike any other system or polling that is always extremely biased.

The energoinformational parameters of *Horus'* single image are greater than those of *The Code of Life's* prime block. There also is something else, some magic, in the image of

Horus. It carries within and projects without the great mysterious power of the ancient culture, which adds indescribable but highly pronounced strength to the new *Code*. Altogether, it makes *The Code of Horus* far more powerful than *The Code of Life*.

Frequency has no upper limit; the Code's potential is limitless. There is no end to more and more powerful Codes, which eventually leads to the discovery and utilization of our inherent abilities to know without tools and heal without doctors and medicines.

I printed one image of Horus on both sides of one page, thus creating *The Code of Horus*. The image's size does not affect its frequency. The Code of Horus generates 300% energy and 10 to the 6000 Power frequency in its free state. It is the same frequency as *The Code of Life'* when it is charged.

When *The Code of Horus* is charged like we charge *The Code of Life*, its energy rises to 700% with 10 to 100.000 Power frequency. I was tempted to measure the energy and frequency of the Infinite Intelligence but found it defies measurement.

Then, disappointment followed. I was not allowed to charge *The Code of Horus* for a reason explained later in the book.

Because of its powerful source of benevolent energy, every home should have a picture of Horus.

Being in the state of peace, oh Infinite Intelligence, I request thy infinite force to destroy all causes inhibiting my body and brain and restore my body and brain to perfect health.

Your Intel-Star energy level must be 175% to use this request.

The Tree of Life came to Egypt in 4 AD. It is a lovely image depicting six life stages, represented by six birds, meaning the life stages are as fleeting as the bird's flight. It has an overall 200% energy level. It also is a beautiful piece of art. Every bird, including the one on the ground on the right side of the Tree, has a different energy level. The one that is on the ground has a 46% energy level. The birds sitting on the tree branches have the following energy levels (from the bottom up) 52%, 80%, 100%, 150%, and 200.

The Code confirms the Tree of Life came to Egypt from the ancient Sumer civilization founded in the Mesopotamia region of the Fertile Crescent situated between the Tigris and Euphrates rivers. While I was trying to find the origins of the Tree of Life, I was led to more discoveries. The original Tree of Life was "created" many years ago. Or was it ever created?

About three million years back, our humanity descended from another civilization on Earth that existed before us. The first people appeared on Earth about 12 million years ago. They came to Earth from the depth of Infinite Intelligence. *The Code* advises human beings were not originated in the depths of Infinite Intelligence. It says humanity exists forever, moving from one energy level to another without a beginning and end. It would be more appropriate to say an Intel-Star exists eternally, moving from one energy level to another, with no beginning and no end. The Infinite Intelligence's descendants "brought" the Tree of Life that exists forever, like Infinite Intelligence and Humanity.

What about our Universe? It looks like Elon Musk guessed it right. The Universe appeared as if by "accident." It has never happened before and will not happen again. It means we live an extraordinary life in the unique place called Earth and have a unique experience that will never occur to humanity again. When the Universe dissolves into nothingness in less than one trillion light-years, humanity in its physical form will also disappear with everything it created. Yet, the Intel-Star will exist forever, keeping the records of our experience.

Fountain of Youth: *The Code of Horus with the Tree of Life System.*

The Code of Horus+ is made of one page with the image of the *Tree of Life* printed on both sides of the page and one page with the image of Horus printed on both sides of the page. I call it *The Code of Horus+* to distinguish it from *The Code of Horus,* created <u>without</u> the *Tree of Life.* I also call it *Fountain of Youth* because, with *The Code of Horus+,* we may restore the body nearly to its youthful condition (some restrictions may apply.)

The Code of Horus+ cannot be charged. In its free state, it has a 10.000% energy level and 10 to the 10 million power frequency. With *The Code of Horus+,* you also will experience greater communications and responses to queries. Only people with a175% and higher energy may use *The Code of Horus+*. However, regardless of the energy level, anyone could keep several copies of *The Code of Horus* (not *The Code of Horus+*) in the fridge, the freezer, and the counters. You are in charge. Consult *The Code.*

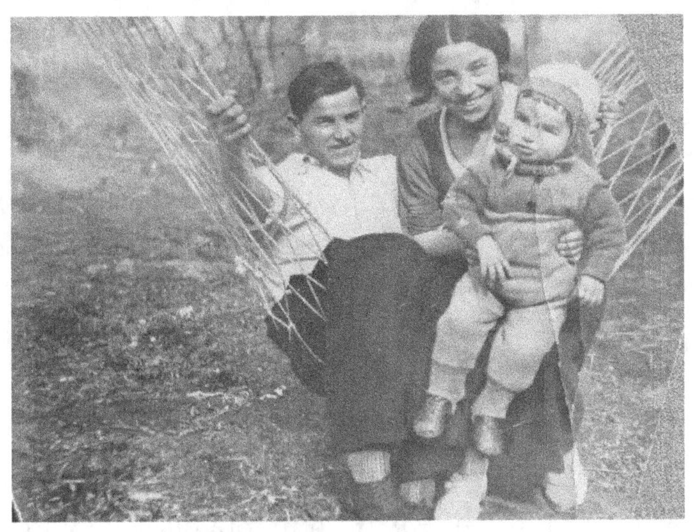

Everything was simple when I was two years old

Mastering simplicity

Information in this chapter and all other chapters is written for people with 52% to 80% Intel-Star energy levels. When your energy is above 80%, adjust it accordingly.

The Code of Life is at the root of Life. With the Simplicity method, we utilize the full power of *The Code* without using tools but using our inherent ability to receive the right knowledge. You must trust yourself. You do not have to trust anyone in the world, but you must trust yourself with no doubts whatsoever. You will know who else you can trust when you have this kind of trust.

We are born self-sufficient and all-knowing. However, our brain does not store any knowledge except the one we put there. Some glands in our brains function as receptors of the boundless field of information stored in the *Infinite Intelligence*. As it was mentioned earlier, *Infinite Intelligence and an Infinite field of knowledge* are the same. Add here Love, and you have a complete picture of the ocean we live in. We could also call it the field of all knowledge. As we grow up, these receptors are getting damaged by pathogens, overwhelmed by misinformation we have been taught is truthful. Thus, we can no longer receive the right knowledge from *Infinite Intelligence*. We accept much wrong, harmful information that is stored in the brain that makes us liarsd, and you already know the consequences

As explained in *Key Points*, to restore our ability to receive true knowledge from the *Infinite Intelligence*, we must raise our Intel-Star energy level to 180%. It is essential to practice watching the mind to help discard misinformation. The higher our Intel-Star energy level, the sounder and greater our accomplishments will be.

Master of simplicity could learn the truth about the person in question, diagnose, do tests, etc., and receive an answer to any inquiry without using the tools. A human being is meant to be independent of the tools, teachers, teachings, doctors, medicines, supplements, and governments.

Such human beings will never hurt anyone, lie, commit fraud, or any crime.

Read a Love poem of your choice. Sit in a chair behind the table; place *The Code* on top of the table in front of you. Put your hands on top of your thighs. Order your left hand to mean No, the right – Yes, or vice versa. Get comfortable. Relax.

Instantly strain your upper arms, and feel a point between the eyes. Relax. Ask your question: "Do I need to restore my vision? <u>Yes or Not</u>?"

Strain your upper arms, and feel the point between the eyes. Relax but keep all three points simultaneously. You may repeat the question or say, "Yes or Not!" Gently keep concentrating on three points. You would feel sensations in one of your hands in a split second. It may be tickling in one hand; one hand could feel heavier or warmer than the other, or it may be just felt while the other – would not. It may be even simpler: your attention will be directed to one of your hands. There certainly will be a pronounced difference between your two hands. A hand that is felt is the answer.

The three points issue is vital to understand. When you are simultaneously feeling all three points, it helps to take attention from everything else, even from your hands, especially – from the mind. When this three-point feeling is established, usually, in one or two seconds, suddenly, you would feel a sensation in one of your hands. The three points are essential when it comes to accuracy.

This method requires almost no time to practice. In my experience, it works like a clock. In the beginning, I was rechecking the result with the Star Pendulum, but only in the very beginning. The results were always the same. It is the simplest method and most comfortable to use. It is also accurate; I would say – precise. To use it, your energy level must be 100% and higher.

This method is superior to the SP because you utilize your inherent ability to know all you wish to know without using tools.

You are born all-knowing. The Simplicity method is as natural as breathing to receive an accurate answer. All you need is confidence and little practice. The Simplicity method verifies our inherent ability to receive the correct answer to every question without tools.

You will be convinced of these methods' accuracy when you become more skillful with the Simplicity Method and The Star Pendulum. Your Biocomputer will tell exactly, for example, how many pushups you need to make at the moment☺

Courtesy of Plentiful Facts

EQUAL LINES

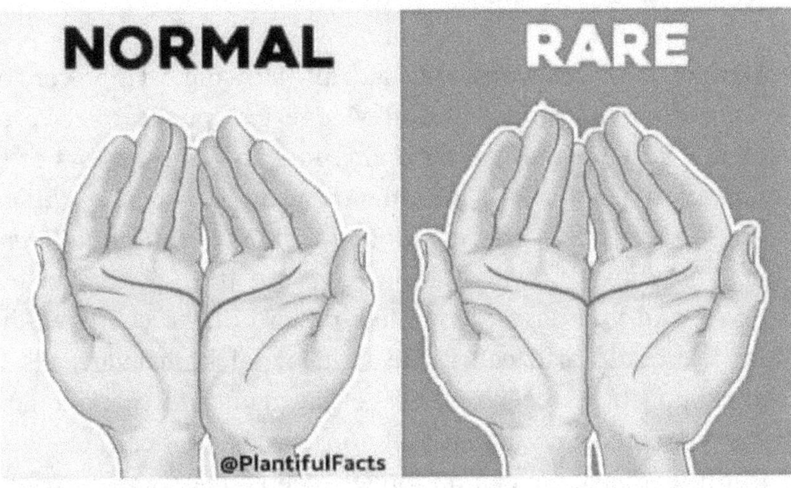

The one most noteworthy line in the palm is located right below the base of the fingers. It's called the heart line. if these lines match up, you have a heart of gold. You are gentle, kinda, and are a source of positive energy. People gravitate to you for support and always find that their favorite moments are with you.

I checked it with *The Code* and found it is accurate. You may use it to determine who is in front of you instantly. If you are proficient with the SP and Simplicity Method, you could evaluate it remotely.

Information in this chapter and all other chapters is written for people with 52% to 80% Intel-Star energy levels. When your energy is above 80%, adjust it accordingly.

The Code of Life is at the root of Life. With the Simplicity method, we utilize the full power of *The Code* without using tools but using our inherent ability to receive the right knowledge. You must trust yourself. You do not have to trust anyone in the world, but you must trust yourself with no doubts whatsoever. You will know who else you can trust when you have this kind of trust.

We are born self-sufficient and all-knowing. However, our brain does not store any knowledge except the one we put there. Some glands in our brains function as receptors of the boundless field of information stored in the *Infinite Intelligence*. As it was mentioned earlier, *Infinite Intelligence and an Infinite field of knowledge* are the same. Add here Love, and you have a complete picture of the ocean we live in. We could also call it the field of all knowledge. As we grow up, these receptors are getting damaged by pathogens, overwhelmed by misinformation we have been taught is truthful. Thus, we can no longer receive the right knowledge from *Infinite Intelligence*. We accept much wrong, harmful information that is stored in the brain that makes us liers, and you already know the consequences

As explained in *Key Points*, to restore our ability to receive true knowledge from the *Infinite Intelligence*, we must raise our Intel-Star energy level to 180%. It is essential to practice watching the mind to help discard misinformation. The higher our Intel-Star energy level, the sounder and greater our accomplishments will be.

Master of simplicity could learn the truth about the person in question, diagnose, do tests, etc., and receive an answer to any inquiry without using the tools. A human being is meant to be independent of the tools, teachers, teachings, doctors, medicines, supplements, and governments.

Such human beings will never hurt anyone, lie, commit fraud, or any crime.

Read a Love poem of your choice. Sit in a chair behind the table; place *The Code* on top of the table in front of you. Put your hands on top of your thighs. Order your left hand to mean No, the right – Yes, or vice versa. Get comfortable. Relax.

Instantly strain your upper arms, and feel a point between the eyes. Relax. Ask your question: "Do I need to restore my vision? Yes or Not?"

Strain your upper arms, and feel the point between the eyes. Relax but keep all three points simultaneously. You may repeat the question or say, "Yes or Not!" Gently keep concentrating on three points. You would feel sensations in one of your hands in a split second. It may be tickling in one hand; one hand could feel heavier or warmer than the other, or it may be just felt while the other – would not. It may be even simpler: your attention will be directed to one of your hands. There certainly will be a pronounced difference between your two hands. A hand that is felt is the answer.

The three points issue is vital to understand. When you are simultaneously feeling all three points, it helps to take attention from everything else, even from your hands, especially – from the mind. When this three-point feeling is established, usually, in one or two seconds, suddenly, you would feel a sensation in one of your hands. The three points are essential when it comes to accuracy.

This method requires almost no time to practice. In my experience, it works like a clock. In the beginning, I was rechecking the result with the Star Pendulum, but only in the very beginning. The results were always the same. It is the simplest method and most comfortable to use. It is also accurate; I would say – precise. To use it, your energy level must be 100% and higher.

This method is superior to the SP because you utilize your inherent ability to know all you wish to know without using tools.

You are born all-knowing. The Simplicity method is as natural as breathing to receive an accurate answer. All you need is confidence and little practice. The Simplicity method verifies our inherent ability to receive the correct answer to every question without tools.

You will be convinced of these methods' accuracy when you become more skillful with the Simplicity Method and The Star Pendulum. Your Biocomputer will tell exactly, for example, how many pushups you need to make at the moment ☺

The Star Pendulum™ (the SP)

It is called the Star Pendulum because people believed it was moved by the stars, i. e., the operator was connected to the stars. The truth is that the SP is moved by the star – our Biocomputer – the entire brain when the mind is quiet.

Indeed, SP is not for everyone because some people "do not have the brain." Only people with an 80% Intel-Star energy level and higher could use the SP. When the Intel-Star level is lower, there will be 80 or more mistakes.

It is essential to raise your energy to a higher level to receive accurate replies. Scientists do not trust the SP because they do not understand why some people receive correct answers to their inquiries, but others err. According to *The Code*, science is two hundred years away from understanding the SP, the Simplicity method, an Intel-Star, energy, and its role in human life. Another factor is a contemporary science has only a 51% energy level.

The SP is a weight of about fifteen grams suspended on a thread so that it can freely swing when you hold the end of the thread with your fingers. The thread should be about two-three inches in length. To create SP, you may use any metal, stone, or glass. They also say material and color do not affect the performance of the pendulum. That is what everyone thinks. However, I found it is essential that the SP has the highest energy level possible. Below, there is an ancient seashell.

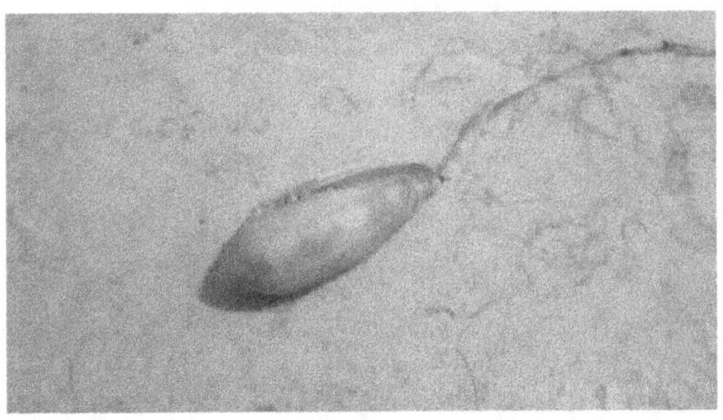

It has 350% energy. However, the energy level of the pendulum does not contribute to the accuracy. Keep in mind your pendulum's shape and weight distribution; it should be evenly weighted.

Choose a quiet place. Sit comfortably at a table. Place a piece of paper on top of the table with a horizontal (-) and a vertical line (+) crossing each other in the middle.

You must first "program" your Biocomputer to work with the SP. I. e., to make your Biocomputer provide the correct answer. Lift the SP by the end of the thread with your forefinger and thumb.

Place your elbow on the table, holding the SP above the paper with two crossing lines. Keep it above the center of the cross. Start programming your Biocomputer by choosing the SP's movement along the vertical line, answering "Yes" and along the horizontal line "No" or "Not."

If the sun was shining, ask, "Is the sun shining?" and lightly push the SP along the horizontal (No) line. If after this light push along the horizontal line, the SP will swing and start moving around, and its final movement would be in the "Yes" direction, you have done it. Your Biocomputer is programmed to move the SP along the vertical line when "Yes" is a correct reply to your inquiry. Repeat the exercise several times with different objects.

Suppose, during the "Yes" programming exercise the SP does not end up moving along the vertical line. In that case, you need to keep practicing until its final movement is in the correct direction.

Do the same with a "No" or "Not" reply along the horizontal line.

The secret is not a secret; it is only practice. Practice with the conviction that you are harmonizing the SP's response with your Biocomputer, which in this case, is a simple command to move along the vertical or horizontal line. The higher is your energy level, the sooner you will receive an accurate reply to every inquiry.

After your successful initial programming, begin practicing with simple questions requiring answers "Yes" or "Not." For example, you may know someone blond. Ask your Biocomputer, "Is this person blond?" You should receive a positive reply.

After asking a question, pay close attention to your arm. You must not influence the SP with your arm, hand, or fingers movement. Be calm and hold a thread very lightly; do not press it. It often happens involuntarily. We tend to "help" the SP move in the direction we want. This trend would become more evident when you diagnose yourself. Therefore, be calm, attentive, and patient. There should be no thoughts or emotions. Calmly concentrate on the SP, keeping your request in the back of your mind. Do not think about the answer that you want to receive.

Before the session with the SP, you must ask the following:

- Any Interference? This means that anything, such as your thoughts, moods, stress or outward energies, noise, etc., is interfering with your work.

The SP must provide you with a negative response.

Then ask:

- "Connected?" It means whether your SP is connected/tuned to your Biocomputer and is ready to work.

The SP must provide you with a positive response.

Our space is saturated with energies of various frequencies. Some flows of energy are strong. You may also happen to be in the geopathogenic zone. Energy movements may also be caused by the sun rising and setting. When you receive a positive reply to the first question, do not attempt to work with the SP, as you will err. Resume your session in ten minutes. You may ask if the interference is internal or external. I have always been receiving a correct reply to this question despite interference.

Sometimes, my SP gave me a runaround when I did not ask the first questions. It would say YES, and when I checked out the answer, it would tell No. If I try to pinpoint some location, the SP would say YES at the particular building, but when I try to confirm it, it would say No. I learned it is a sure sign of some interference, outer or inner. More than often, it was an emotional interference. In this case, I would recite a poem and resume my work within a few minutes. I found external interference happens rarely.

After becoming confident and experienced in getting the right answer, you may check your answers by pushing the SP in the wrong direction. For example, you know this person is blond. Ask, "Is this person blond?" Wait a second. If the SP does not move, push/move it lightly in the wrong (negative) direction. It will start moving in the direction it was pushed, but then, without any influence on your part, it will swing in the opposite direction, which means you received the right (positive) response: the person is blond indeed. Carefully watch for the tendency to "help" the SP move in your desired direction. Keep practicing with similar questions. When you "gain speed," you will be able to receive answers about the level (percentages) of different qualities of any person on earth, alive or dead. "Is this person honest?" "Does Peter truly love me? ☺ Remember the rules.

Learn to let the SP fly free. Push it lightly along the horizontal line and unnoticeably influence this horizontal flight. It must feel like the SP is flying on its own. It may move in circles, right and left, and circle again to answer your question. Make sure there is no interference. Eventually, the SP will steady itself in one direction, which is the answer. Unless you are the SP genius, meaning your energy level is close to 200%, it may take two to three days of practice before you can fly it free. When you get a feeling of the free flight, you will also notice that the SP is moving as if by itself and tends to increase speed when providing you with the right answer.

After initial questions, when you want to know your weight, ask, "What is my weight?" and lightly move the SP in the negative direction while saying with every two-three swings, Fifty-two, Fifty-four, Fifty-six…. At some point, as if by itself, the SP would change the direction to the "Yes" vertical movement. It is your answer. Ask if the number is correct. It is a super easy one to check!

Only when your energy level is below 100%, use printed The Coe of Life:

When asking a question, hold the SP <u>over</u> *The Code of Life*. It will ensure the accuracy of the reply. After you raise your energy and gain experience, you will not need to keep *The Code* close to yourself, as explained in The Code of Life Communications and System of Health.

Read a poem (see: *Addendum*), then ask the two preliminary questions ("Interference?", "Contact?"), then – your inquiry. You may make several inquiries at just a minute or two intervals, but if you get out of your chair even for a few minutes, you will have to ask the two preliminary questions again before your next inquiry. Ideally, ask the two initial questions before each query.

Hold the SP's thread gently, letting your Biocomputer direct it, not your fingers or arm (a metal ring at the end of the thread may be helpful). Be relaxed and thoughtless. It comes with a bit of practice. Your arm will move following your Biocomputer's orders, yet this movement is so subtle you can hardly notice it. If you are aware of your hand's motion and your fingers, your mind is interfering. It must be felt as if the SP is flying by itself. So, let it fly free and enjoy its flight.

You can check the accuracy of every reply you receive. It is a simple procedure. Ask, "Using a scale from 0 to 100%, how accurate is the reply I just received?" Let the SP have a free horizontal fly while saying 50%... 60%...70%... 90%... 95%... 98%... at some point, the SP would move, tend to move, or swing towards the vertical direction; it is the answer. With time, you would notice an almost invisible change in the SP's movement. Do not be anxious; this time will come soon. You will be pleasantly surprised at how soon it will come. For example, the answer is 67%. Check it out, asking, "Is it more than 67%?" When the reply is negative, count again, starting with 55%. After about thirty days of working with the SP on and off, a reader sent me this message:

"YURI!!!! I have started TODAY!!!! The SP was moving freely. It was moving in circles in the past, but now it went up and down for YES and left to right for NO very clearly. I asked 2 test questions.

"I don't have diabetes, and I don't need red meat, and my husband is not cheating on me (that was the question I was afraid to ask; you knew that something was bothering me)."

When I checked the above replies, they were all correct. You would master the SP much sooner when practicing <u>every day</u>.

The SP works harmoniously with our Biocomputer (the brain). You must turn off your conscious mind and wordlessly concentrate on action consisting of two parts. First, formulate a question like "What is the PH of my liver's tissue?" or "Is it beneficial to invest in Cannabis $1000 with (the name of the company) recommended by The Motley Fool?" knowing that you are programming your Biocomputer with these questions. By the way, most recommendations of this kind are fraud ☺ Exceptions are rare. Cannabis is 95% harmful. Even when used as a painkiller, cancer is its side effect.

With the SP, we can receive answers virtually to any question: the quality of food and automobile, the "quality" of the relationship, politics, finances, geopathogenic zone, and the life resource. In addition, we could check our decisions, diagnose our state of health, the health of any human being, animal, and plant located on the other side of the Earth, and much more.

You wish to know if an object/product you want is good for you. Not all that we want is good for us. Also, some things that are good for one person may harm another. The Biocomputer will analyze your request, direct muscles to move the SP, and provide you with a correct answer. The simple secret is letting your Biocomputer do the job, not the mind.

Another use for your SP is learning more about the foods you ingest and how they affect your body. Say you have an unopened jar of honey. Even in sealed glass, plastic, even metal, or wood container, the SP will be able to tell you if you need it.

You will soon come to the point when you are calmly watching your arm unnoticeably directed, not by the mind. You will realize it is a complex, benevolent, and intelligent system – your entire brain– your Biocomputer.
When filing a request, choose from several beautiful poems in the end of the book, the one that is close to your heart. Reciting a poem will bring you closer to the state of True Love. However, you need not recite a poem when your energy level is above 130%. I love these poems and repeat them often.

Adopted concepts and dogmas will cause you to err. When free, we have no adopted doctrines, dogmas, or concepts, and we hardly make mistakes.

Michael believes in reincarnation. He errs when he wants the answer on the subject, even indirectly related to reincarnation. It happens because any belief is checked against the Truth. Psychological conflict is created, indicating something is wrong when our belief does not match the Truth, resulting in stress and error. The Truth does not tolerate lies, dogmas, and concepts; every concept is artificial, and every belief system is erroneous. There are no exceptions.

When there is no knowing mind, there are no concepts. Forget, dismiss, and set aside everything you learned. Let the mind be stark naked. Only then would the Infinite Intelligence lead you as it leads little crab in the following story, leading every insect, bird, and animal.

This story took place shortly after I discovered *The Code*. At the time, I always kept it in my backpack. I was on a tiny beach at Mt. Argentario, Italy, charging *The Code* to dissolve calcium deposits in my Inner Carotid vein, when a man approached me. He was in his seventies, tall and slim, a Russian tourist.

"I see you are working with the Pendulum," he said casually. "I heard about it, wanted to learn it, but could not get the right information." His English was quite good. "Where did you learn such good English," I smiled. "I was sailing on traders all my life," he smiled in return, "and I love English." We talked for a couple of minutes, and then he said, "I want to ask you a small favor." I nodded encouragingly. "There is some problem with my passport. Maybe you could try and figure it out with your pendulum." "Sure," I said. "Why do you think there is a problem?"

"Maybe it is something else, but I noticed when I am in my room that I am coughing every time I have this passport near me. And my friend also starts coughing when she comes over to visit." "You are not coughing now," I said. "You're right," he replied, "I noticed it happens only in a closed space, like a hotel room." He gave me the passport, and I checked it out with my SP, asking if there was any problem. Immediately the SP began to move up and down. There was a problem. What was it? My next question was how serious the problem was. The SP kept moving with increasing speed. "Is it something dangerous," That was my next question. It was affirmative. I checked the degree of danger. It was 99%.

Instinctively, I dropped the passport on the sand before me as I realized there was something terrible in my hand. The man, Maxim Savin, was his name, noticed my reaction. "Is it bad?" He asked. "It is bad," I replied. "We have to figure out what it is," I murmur to myself, "And we will."

"I do not need to hold your passport in my hands to figure out the problem." Maxim was about to pick up the passport, but I stopped him: "Please, leave it there until we are done." To my next question, if the passport was treated with some chemicals, the SP's reply was affirmative. I kept asking and finally got the answer: it was treated with Strontium 90.

Maxim was shocked. I determined that five layers of foil would keep him out of danger.

"You see, Maxim," I said when we parted, "Once you learn how to work with the SP, you will never have a similar problem and other problems and become your best doctor." "Would you, please, help me with it," he was almost pleading. I nodded. "I am about to finish *The Code of Life Communications and System of Health.* I'll send it to you in July."

A few days later, I suddenly decided to diagnose myself. I found no traces of Strontium 90. Yet, there were pathogens in my left lung and aorta. I traced it back to my encounter with Maxim and discovered the cause. It was fear, fear of contamination.

Interestingly, Maxim also had pathogens in the lungs and liver. Fear caused it. I taught him how to eliminate it. One month later, I remotely diagnosed him and found no traces of Strontium 90 in his body.

Fear can be deadly. It is at the root of all negative emotions and is often the cause of health problems. Whenever there is a surge of fear, transform it into Love.

Be patient, and start with simple things. Pay attention to how you phrase your questions, as one word included/excluded or mispronounced could swerve your results. Double-check your answers.

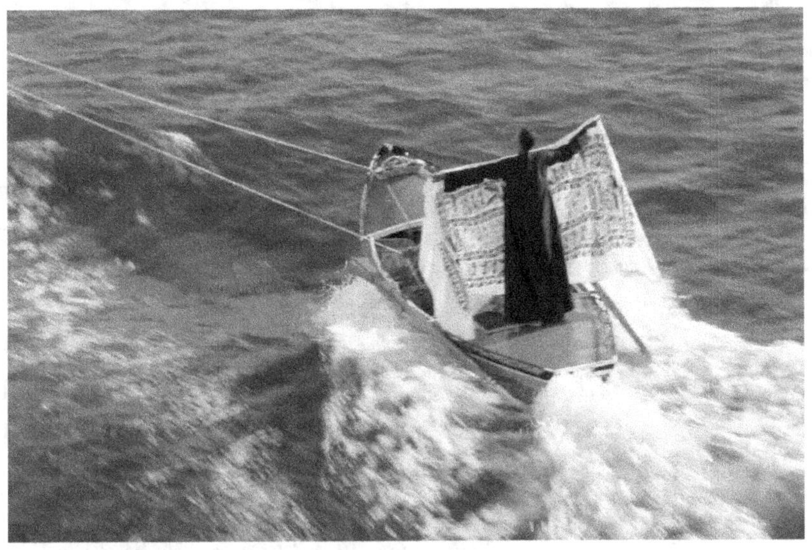

A Nile River salesman in Egypt

Key points

Information in this chapter is written for people with 52% to 80% Intel-Star energy levels. When your energy is above 80%, adjust it accordingly, like using *The Code of Horus* and destroying the causes instead of particular reasons: pathogens, deposits, pesticides, etc. However, in some cases, while eliminating the causes, you may also need to destroy specific pathogen(s), restore genes, and dissolve deposits.

Tests. We made many tests in California and conducted tests remotely to destroy pesticides, hormones, pathogens, and other foreign matter in vegetables and fruits with *The Code of Life*. Various products were placed on the table in Yaroslavl, Russia. A picture of the product was displayed (it is optional because the test can be made without a picture, and without the computer) on the computer screen in California.

1. In California, we determined what foreign matter (pesticides, hormones, pathogens, etc.) was present in the tested product. Both operators recorded and verified the result (in Yaroslavl and California). Upon comparing records, they appear the same: pesticides and pathogens in tested products.

2. In California, we charged *The Code of Life* with the request to destroy pesticides and pathogens in the product displayed on the screen:

   Being in the state of Love, Oh, Love! I request thy Infinite Power to charge The Code of Life with the full strength of thy energy to destroy pesticides and Pathogens in Onion, Banana, and Potato. Thank you! Thank you! Thank you! We kept charging *The Code* for 30 seconds.

3. Again, we remotely determined if any foreign matter (in this case, pesticides and pathogens) was still present in the tested product. Both operators recorded and verified the result (in Yaroslavl and California).

Upon comparing records, they appeared the same: all foreign matter was destroyed in the tested product.

We were using the SP in the tests to verify the results. Unfortunately, the energy-deficient scientific community does not yet accept the SP. We attempted to do formal lab tests for more than one year, experiencing disbelief and a rigid ignorant attitude. The destruction of parasites and chemicals with The Code of Life is beyond the comprehension of the professional mind.

The Power of Love. True Love *(Love with a capital "L") is kindness, compassion, understanding, and acceptance. Love is at the root of every human experience of love.*

There is often confusion about the word "acceptance." It means accepting the world the way it is and people as they are without judging and trying to change them while being in a state of inner peace, regardless of what we see. Our energy level determines our ability to employ Love's power.

The higher our energy level, the higher the frequency, and the sooner we accomplish the task. When our energy level is low, we need to charge *The Code of Life* more to achieve the same result. When the energy level is below 52%, we cannot employ *The Code* (some exceptions apply). The reason is that a person's energy level of 52% is a "threshold of goodness." Beyond this threshold, our energy is no longer benevolent, and *The Code* has high-level benevolent energy.

The absence of the necessary energy is destructive as the lower frequency energy, with its longer ways, begins to take over. The lower our energy level, the lower its frequency, the longer its waves, and the more damaging it becomes. When the low-energy person enters the room, watch your emotions. A low-energy person can give you a bad feeling in the pit of your stomach, make you cringe, and lose your emotional balance.

Contrary to popular belief, organic farming does use pesticides. Over a hundred fertilizers and inputs (pesticides, insecticides, or fungicides) are authorized by organic farming regulations in Europe and the United States.

Pesticides approved for organic farming include neem oil, made from the neem tree, and pyrethrin, made from chrysanthemum plants. A few synthetic chemicals are also allowed in organic agriculture. Examples include copper sulfate, alcohols, chlorine products, hydrogen peroxide, and soaps.

In addition to communications and healing properties, *The Code of Life* has many other uses, including nearly instant rendering harmless pesticides, hormones, pathogens, and heavy metals in foodstuffs. To accomplish it, charge and place *The Code of Life* in the refrigerator overnight, and all food will become truly organic.

The Code of Life is a natural cleanser; unlike a commercial organic procedure, it uses high-frequency energy for cleansing.

You may have three additional *Codes of Life* (one in the freezer) and two permanently set in your fridge. Charge them once in 24 hrs. without taking them out or opening the door.

An average American has about 62% energy level. Our energy level should be 65% and higher to efficiently use *The*

Code of Life. You may still use the system while having a lower energy level. The procedure would take a long time or forever. Raise your energy level.

Elevating energy level. What is the difference between you and Buddha? There is only one difference: your mind is clogged with teachers, teachings, dogmas, gods, and cultural drivel; Buddha's mind was nearly stark naked. The "Spiritual" industry complicated this issue, but it is as simple as a whistle.

Drop teachers; they are all but egotistic fraud. What is a teacher when there is nothing to teach? The US teachers' average Intel-Star energy level, including those from the East, is a disastrous 8%. Many of them are violating the laws of nature. Drop all teachings, for there are no helpful teachings whatsoever. Every Eastern teaching is rooted in the Vedas and Upanishads. With their energy levels below 10%, these two sources embody utter ignorance, a total distortion of the Truth.

Most teachings, tools, and practices were imported from the east, with its population having an overall 13% Intel-Star energy level. In India, over 50% of the male population has an Intel-Star energy level below 15%, resulting from millenniums' adherence to falsehood. Everything coming from there is damaging, even detrimental to one's health.

Drop all cultural drivel with its news and entertainment of all kinds. The US news media has an overall Intel-Star energy level of 8%, which means fake news. TV shows, movies, anchors, so-called "celebrities," "stars," producers, and directors are poisoning you with their overall disastrous 6% energy level.

When you drop it all, your energy level will jump to 100% and higher, and you will see the light of day. You will make the right decisions and live a truly happy and fulfilling life. Of course, you may still get irritated, emotional, or even angry, but it will be short-lived and will not leave a trace of negativity in the subconscious.

Though the above method is the most efficient way to raise your Intel-Star energy level, the following helps make the subconscious final polishing, cleaning it of the past negative traces. Among benefits of the high energy level, is almost instant healing process. For example, you got older and got high blood sugar level. If your energy level is a 190%, you may normalize it instantly with a simple request:
Oh, Love, I request to normalize my blood sugar level. And it will be normal.

Elevating Intel-Star's energy level by eliminating the influence of negativity of the past.

The world of nature, animals, the Universe, and human beings is the paradise world of Oneness. However, human beings have been endowed with minds. I guess someone up there made a mistake. Look at animals. When there is no human interference, animals do not get ill. They do not have a mind; they are in a state of Oneness and led by Infinite Intelligence, like the world of nature is led by Infinite Intelligence.

So far, I guessed but did not discover why we have minds.

The human mind divides Oneness into two worlds by creating a low-energy/frequency world with low-energy people. This world has been created because many children are not raised with Love. How this trend started is another puzzle.

Indeed, our negative past creates a major problem in our way to Peace and Happiness in the Paradise world of Oneness because it obstructs Love and negatively influences our decisions. We have tested the Elevating positive energy level technique. It is similar to the original Transformation method described in my books; it is also more comfortable to employ and check the progress. Using the Elevating Intel-Star energy level technique after dumping all teachers and teachings will eliminate every trace of the past negativity.

Begin with determining how much negativity remains in your subconscious archive out of 100% of the negativity accumulated during the first ten years of your life.

1. How much negativity remains in my subconscious archive, considering all the negativity I have accumulated in my first ten years to be a 100%?

2. (Optional) Let the Star Pendulum move freely along the horizontal line while counting with every couple of swings "5", "10", "15", end so on. The Star Pendulum would tend to move toward the vertical line. It may be a very light movement. You would instantly notice the Star Pendulum's almost unnoticeable tendency to change direction and recheck it with practice. Let us say it is 26%. The amount of remaining negativity is not essential. It demonstrates you have carried through life negativity obtained in your first ten years and reminds you of your inspirations, dreams, and decisions that were often sabotaged by this negativity and the negativity accumulated in later years.

Every negative event generates negative low-frequency energy that damages the organs and systems. It is the prime reason why stress must be avoided. When the event is intense, like in child abuse, it would also disorient the child's genes in the brain and the genome of neurons – carriers of the memory traces.

 The damage opens the "door" for pathogens (Protozoa and Fungus) to enter and set in neurons. A damaged genome and parasites will cause neurons to malfunction, creating a negative field that would adversely influence the child's life and as a grown-up. Pathogens must be destroyed and the genome restored to resume neurons' normal activity.

In case of a mild adverse event, our immune system will do its job by eliminating pathogens and repairing the damage. File the request with the Power of Love.

> *Being in the state of Love, Oh, Love! I request thy Infinite Power to charge my Code of Life with the full strength of thy energy to destroy Protozoa and Fungus and restore genes in the neurons affected by adverse situations in the first ten years of my life.*

When your energy level is below 80%, keep charging *The Code* for 30 seconds.

> The Biocomputer focuses *The Code*'s high frequency energy on the target and destroys what we have programmed to destroy. We are using not some outside force but the high-frequency energy we label Love, multiplied by our charge many a hundred times. With pathogens destroyed, the genome restored, and neurons healed, the negative influence is dissolved. Thus, we are reducing the amount of subconscious negativity and intensifying the frequency of our energy.

Repeat this process every ten years of your life. You could narrow it down to every five, four, one year, or even one month. The shorter the period you choose, the more effective is cleansing.

Afterward, verify there is no negativity left in your subconscious archive in the corresponding period of life. Repeat when it is necessary. Depending on your energy level, it may be required to repeat the process.

Remember to have two and a half hour breaks between requests. Depending on your energy level, a pause may be shorter.

The Intel-Star energy level can drop quickly

When you live with Love, you make fewer mistakes, and your Intel-Star energy will rise. However, when you transgress the laws of nature and do something wrong, your Intel-Star energy level will drop. Following is a tragic true story.

Sergey went to the war when he was nineteen. His Intel-Star energy level was 170%. Sergey's infinite trust in Pendant was the only reason for the Intel-Star energy level. His mother gave it to him. Inside the Pendant, there was an old yellowish piece of paper with three words written in old Russian letters, saying You Are Safe.

"This Pendant is magical." Said the mother. "It saved your great grandfather in the war with Turks, and then – your father's life in the Civil war."

Of course, it was not magic but a high energy level that saved Sergey's ancestors: their Intel-Star energy level was around 170%.

"I don't remember how many companies I have changed," Sergey said, "People died around me, but I got only a scratch on my arm in five years of this bloody war."

When I met Sergey, his Intel-Star energy level was only 47%. After the war, he became a police officer, and he hated his job. He was drinking. He showed me his Pendant. "I believed in it with all my heart. It proved its magic in three wars, and it saved my life," he said and hung the Pendant back on his neck. "Now there is no war," he continued, "It lost its magic… Now it is helpless."

The power was certainly not in the Pendant; it was in the strength of Sergey's faith caused by the high Intel-Star energy level. Sergey's wife died of cancer. Their daughter was married and lived in London. Sergey was a very lonely man. Two years later, I was told, Sergey jumped to his death from the ten-story balcony. He dreaded heights.

Shortly before Sergey died, his energy level dropped to 21%. After the war, Sergey's Intel-Star energy level was 60%. Many causes were inhibiting his energy level. These causes had to be eliminated, but who would know at that time how to eradicate causes and raise the energy level?

Sergey put all his trust in the Pendant. That trust temporarily raised his energy level very high, but his negative past – the leading cause of our problems, was not cleaned. There were other causes. If Sergey maintained his trust, he would have lived a life of happiness, regardless of circumstances that were far not as severe as in the war. He did not. His invisible past took over.

Infinite Intelligence

Bees and ants, birds, animals, all nature, our world, the universe, and humanity live in the ocean of the *Infinite Intelligence,* which is the *Infinite Field of Knowledge. Infinite Intelligence* guides every living being except mindful human beings. It is freely accessible by the person with 175% energy. It is "accidentally" accessible by everyone else when they "accidentally" happen to "fall" into a high-frequency range (revelations, discoveries). The frequency of the *Infinite Intelligence* cannot be determined.

In the brain, several glands (frontal lobe, hypophysis, pineal gland, vascular plexus of the side ventricle, and two others) provide us with access to the *Infinite Intelligence.* Information in the *Infinite Intelligence* is only 100% true. The *Infinite Intelligence* does not contain information created by people, no matter how truthful it may seem. Information created by the mind cannot be 100% true as the mind is not perfect.

The mind does not make discoveries. Discoveries are made at the time when the mind, exhausted with a search, falls quiet. At that moment an Intel-Star energy level may rise to 175% and higher, and we receive the information we seek. The mind gets the credit.

In most people, the receptors are blocked due to medical issues, false knowledge, and pathogens. Thus, the blockage is shutting down the ability to receive data from *Infinite Intelligence.* Unfortunately, it is something that Medical Science does not deal with, as no technology exists to monitor this issue.

A state of peace is the necessary condition for contacting the *Infinite Intelligence.* Discoveries are made, and revelations are received only in this state. Whatever we accept as being true, our Biocomputer equates to the *Infinite Intelligence* with what is truly right. We call it our judge within, but we do not know what part of the brain plays the role of the judge within. It is not Intel-Star either.

The Code confirms that false information is still compared to the information stored in the *Infinite Intelligence* despite the receptors being closed. I have not yet learned the mechanics of it. But it is how psychological conflict is created when we believe in something that is not true. It leads to irritation and stress. The *Infinite Intelligence* and our Biocomputer do not compromise, but the mind is compromising all the time by believing deceitful things being truthful, as happened, for example, with Einstein's theory of relativity and religion.

One of the reasons society and religion failed to improve human beings and make the world better is an overwhelming amount of false information fed to the masses as truthful. However, the temporary setbacks cannot halt or reverse the evolution's upward trend. We are born perfect. We have everything necessary to create a life of health, happiness, and success. We have the power to make our world a Paradise. To achieve it, we do not need external help; we do not need teachers and teachings. All we need is Love, to live by the energy of Love and higher energies. We need to keep raising our Intel-Star energy level. Nature presented us with *The Code of Life* to unclutter our inherent ability to be our best doctors and teachers and make our world a beautiful place.

Celebrities and Theft of energy

Jake and Jill

My life changed after I discovered *The Code of Life.* It has changed for the better in every aspect except for my friends. Living alone in the Sierra Mountains, I did not socialize and had only a few friends. It was disappointing when I had to lose a friend. It usually happened when I would discover my friend had a low energy level. A dialogue would follow the discovery, and, suddenly, we are poles apart.

Jake and his wife, Jill, loved my books. They came to visit me in the mountains. I came down several times to see them in Santa Barbara. Our relationship was a warm mutual understanding until I published *The Code of Life Communications and System of Health.* Jake said he did not understand it but could not explain why.

We kept exchanging letters. Suddenly, Jake said that I had changed and not for the better. Indeed, I have changed; with *The Code,* my posts became more revealing and direct as my high energy level made me see events and people through and through.

In one of my letters, I mentioned Jill's high 87% Intel-Star energy level. "I don't know about Jill being high energy level." Replied Jake. I saw he meant physical energy. "I think the opposite. She does not DO much all day - she watches TV, will not consider working, and has had a headache for YEARS. I am worried about her. When we met, she relied on me for EVERYTHING and stopped developing herself. Now she acts as if she is somewhat intellectually crippled. So sad. I started chanting with her in the morning for ten minutes, thinking it would help raise her life energy. But I think she doesn't WANT to raise it - I think she's scared to go out in the world - she's used to being beautiful and having the world come to her. I think she would be willing to try *The Code.* Thank you for thinking of us, Yuri. Love."

That letter stirred some strange feelings and made me investigate why a lovely Jill I knew became this way. It did not take me long to guess the puzzle. If you read the book, you would know a simple way to determine a person's low energy level is to offer *The Code of Life Communications and System of Health.* When the energy level is low, the offer is rejected. It was Jake's attitude. To my great surprise, Jake had only an 11% energy level. It was a shocking disappointment! It was also the key to Jill's puzzle.

Jake's low energy was causing Jill's sad state. Its long waves' bashing power has disoriented genes in several glands of Jill's brain, letting fungus and viruses invade the Paraterminal gyrus and Parietooccipital sulcus glands of the brain, as well as the Great cerebral vein (of Galen). Also, Jake was unknowingly feeding on Jill's energy because, like anyone with a low energy level, he was instinctively trying to raise it by sucking out other people's energy to be as far as possible from "zero" or the point of death.

I told Jake the truth and suggested reading the book to Jill as her English was not good enough. I also offered to send *The Code* and make the request for Jill. I have never heard from Jake again.

Without your knowledge, some of your friends, relatives, and people you know and do not know may have been unintentionally feeding on your energy. The culprits may include your teachers, managers, celebrities, friends, and others. The most potent "vampire" of all is your TV screen. Some people have access to the idiot box in the bedroom, restroom, and kitchen in the palm of their hand, which signifies insecurity, inability to enjoy themselves, and running away from themselves. Throw it all out. Every time you view the idiot box, it bombards you with an average of 60% negative energy.

When meeting some people for the first time, you may suddenly feel heaviness, emptiness, and discomfort, even when the person you meet appears to be a pleasant individual. It is especially true with people violating the laws of nature in their private lives. Usually, these are the signs that the low-energy individual is sucking your energy. When you wish to know if someone is feeding on your energy, relax in a chair and use the Simplicity method. Ask your Biocomputer, "Is George feeding on my energy, Yes or Not?" Instantly, you will know.

Some of your favorite celebrities may not be as beautiful people as they are trying to present themselves. Great talent, too often, is deceptive. That's Hollywood with its 6% energy level. It is powerful weaponry – a health-damaging "entertainment" system.

Here are some actors' energy levels: George Clooney 17%; Britney 17%; Tom Hanks 9%; Marlon Brando 9%; Clark Gable 11%. An interviewer once told Gary Grant (17%), "Everybody would like to be Gary Grant," Grant is said to have replied, "So would I." He was right because having only a 17% energy level, he never was the man we wanted to be. Whoopi Goldberg 43%; Jane Fonda 17%; Natalie Wood 13%.

These actors seem to have everything one could dream about, except Love and Happiness, for Love is nearly dead below 50% of the energy level; it is dead below 40%.

These people also are destroyers. Whether dead or alive, when you watch their films, they bombard you with their powerful long waves, causing physical and psychological harm. So be aware and raise your shield of Love whenever you watch them. Knowing the truth, why would you ever watch them? Concentrate on yourself and watch your mind. It is far more entertaining than watching energy-deficient waste of humanity.

To cut off the energy thieves (you may use the SP or not):

1. Ask the SP, "How much energy is sucked by other people and the idiot box from my daily energy supply?" Do not be surprised when you get a number 50% and higher. Some people may lose up to 95% of their daily energy supply and go to bed exhausted.

2. In the Addendum, choose a poem you will use with your request to cut off the energy channels with people feeding on your energy. Trust your intuition about how many times you have to recite it if you did not yet master the SP. Five recitals usually are sufficient.

3. It is <u>not necessary to charge</u> *The Code* with this request. Just place your hands on top of it.

Being in the state of Love, Oh, Love! I request thy Infinite Power cut off all energoinformational channels with people feeding on my energy (including so and so, name people you know).

After filing your request, check your energy level. Repeat at least once a week, and more often when meeting many people.

Always check the energy level of all items that come your way, including cultural, religious, and political things/writings/artifacts, because their low energy could invalidate your work and cause damage. Pay attention to how culture, politics, and religion are trying, by any means, to infiltrate human life. Eradicate or neutralize their influence with requests.

You do not need to check out anything religious because it all has damaging Intel-Star energy levels below 20%.

German Swine in WWII: an overall 17% Intel-Star energy level. It is a powerful demonstration of what deficient energy half-humans can do to others.

In 1997 Chuck Rapoport and I were writing *Stalin*, a five-part miniseries for the CBS Television network. At that time, I had the most horrible experience in my life. I spent many hours in the archive of UCLA, which had a wealth of authentic material on the USSR and WWII.

I came across two pictures from the German archive, captured by the US military at the end of WWII. In one picture, women (87% Intel-Star energy level) walked along a lonely dirt road lined up with leafless trees sticking their bare branches into a grey sky. A bunch of German swine (13% Intel-Star energy level) with guns at the ready accompanied the gloomy crowd. It was an early morning of late fall, and Germans were all wearing heavy overcoats; the pigs hated cold. But the women were all naked!

In the other picture, naked women were lining up the age of the deep trench with bodies at the bottom; some stretched, some curled in death. In the SS lieutenant uniform, a young

German swine commanded the bunch of German rats with rifles aiming at the women. Some bodies were seen in midair, and others about to fall -- murdered.

Recently, medical science discovered something that Tibetan monks new for thousands of years: when physical death happens with the heart stopped, the brain keeps on living for about twenty minutes longer. Tibetan monks called this state Bardo, or after death state. In the past only three persons with incredibly high Intel-star energy level of 350%were able to come back and describe what was taking place in Bardo. These people were living in different centuries, but their accounts were all the same. Depending on their Intel-Star energy levels, people in Bardo state were having different experiences, ranging from pleasant to horrible. Those with a low Intel-Star energy levels are people who hurt others, cheating, lying, believing in a lie, violating the lows of nature. These people were having bad to worst experience. People with   Intel-Star energy levels above the threshold of 52% were having good to pleasant experience. It is from this Bardo state Christianity created ideas of hell and paradise, adding artificial comments.

I do not have the original pictures, but here is one I found on the Web. Intel-Star's energy level of the swine is 9%. The women in the trench have an overall 145% energy level. From the time immemorial, the low-energy pigs have been murdering good people and, usually, were getting away with murders. Nevertheless, all of the murderers of all time are brutally tortured/cleansed in the after-death state called Bardo. Does it make it easier for these women to die?

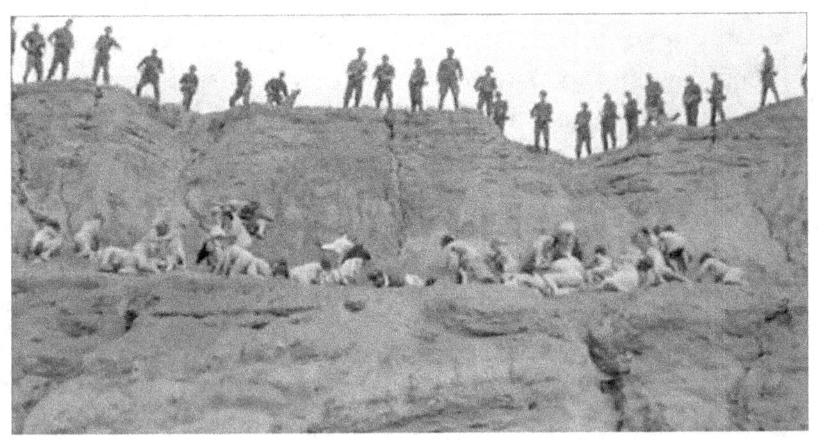

Look at this filthy German swine, a vomit in human form. The German pigs murdered over three million civilians in Ukraine alone during WWII.

Ukraine welcomed fascists because it was treated badly by the fraudulent soviet regime. In the beginning of the Soviet Revolution, on orders of the grand-murderer Lenin, Ukraine was suffocated by hunger with three million people dead. Plus, murdering of the resistance. Ukraine never forgot it. It believed the Germans will free them from Soviet chains. But Hitler was utter stupid and perverted fanatic idiot. He added Ukraine to his death list of blacks and homosexuals. The terrible German crimes were never punished the way they should have been punished. 80% of this rotten military swine were Catholics, but not even one murderer was excommunicated. Catholic church welcomed Hitler, and a fraudulent Catholic Pope wrote a welcoming letter to "Glorious Fuhrer."

When Hitler came to power, the German nation had overall 17% Intel-Star energy. The German military had a 16% Intel-Star energy level. The Germans did not learn a thing from the lessons of WWI. Today, the average German Intel-Star energy level is a deficient 35% which is the world's lowest. People with this low level cannot be trusted and must be carefully watched as they remain the world's treacherous aggressive crowd.

Pictures, books, and figurines are often sources of destructive low energy, especially those depicting fraudulent politicians and religious personalities "dead" or alive. I use quotation marks because many religious characters did not die as they have never been. A lie creates inner conflict because a lie contradicts the Truth.

One of the reasons children do not like school is because of pictures of deceitful politicians on the walls and lies spelled in schoolbooks. Children intuitively feel lies and reject lies.

I remember how exhausted I was after visiting the Pushkin Museum in Moscow, which I loved. The museum has many old religious paintings and statues.

Do you have pictures hanging on the walls? Examine them. They may be a source of low energy. If yes, neutralize its influence. Your energy level must be at least 80%. It is not necessary to charge *The Code*.

Being in the state of Love, Oh Love, I request thy infinite power to wipe out negativity from my pictures and books.

The Code of Life is built with zeros arranged in a specific pattern printed on paper. We cannot verbalize the pattern's meaning, but we know it generates energy with a frequency of ten to the 56 power. We also know this energy is beneficial. It is the same with the written word, with the difference that we know the content and meaning here.

The high-energy people wrote the original Bible with an astounding 99% energy level. Over the years, the Church destroyed all copies of that book. The second version of the Bible had 41% energy, and a contemporary Bible created in the eleven century has 5% energy.

<u>All spiritual</u> books have a very low energy level.

Novels you would not allow to read your 13-year-olds must be thrown out. If you read these books, there must be something wrong with you.

Predictions/Prophecies

With *The Code of Life,* you receive accurate information on anything past and present because the past is written in stone. The present is becoming the past every instant. We cannot change the past; the aware mind can eliminate the influence of the negative past. Diagnosis and healing happen in the present; this data is always accurate.

All predictions and prophecies are pure nonsense. They may be accurate only at the forecast time; they may indeed be wrong an instant later. Nostradamus had an 86% energy level, which grossly erred his predictions when they were made.

Thus, any "prophesy" regarding events in humanity's future is speculation of the prophesy-fabricator. Do not attempt to predict the future. There are always exceptions. Rockefeller insisted he was "bound to be wealthy" and "I would live until I am a hundred years old." He fulfilled both predictions. One may successfully predict things about himself when they have an unwavering belief in their prophecy. Some people's minds are dense like logs with deficient energy levels. Because these people rarely change, their future can be predicted to a degree, including how they will die.

Statistically, people with energy below 12% do not die from natural causes; their brains and bodies are destroyed by the long energy waves that cause cancer and similar diseases.

Everything about us is subject to constant change: environment, relationships, diet, and bricks may fall on our heads, ending up our life along with inquiries☺ When your energy level is 80%, and more, you may ask *The Code,* "What is my life's resource?" and receive accurate information. The data would be correct only for the time of the request. It may change an instant later.

There is a flood of videogames "that predict your future with "insane accuracy." No game or a pack of cards of any kind can predict anything. Advertisers are simply lying; they use one coincidence or another to justify their lies.

The Tarot, Numerology, anything invented by people claiming it predicts the fu**ture – your future – is an outright lie. Nothing created by human** beings could make an accurate prediction, including scriptures. People with low Intel-Star energy levels create this low-energy stuff. The low-energy creations can only mislead. They are disastrous when it comes to a forecast.

Someone with at least 195% energy level could make accurate predictions with *The Code of Horus+* and *The Star,* an almost two million-year-old tree fossil with a 1000% energy level. Like the original *Code of Life, The Code of Horus+* and *The Star* are gifts of nature; no human being has created them. Today, man is incapable of creating systems with such high energy levels.

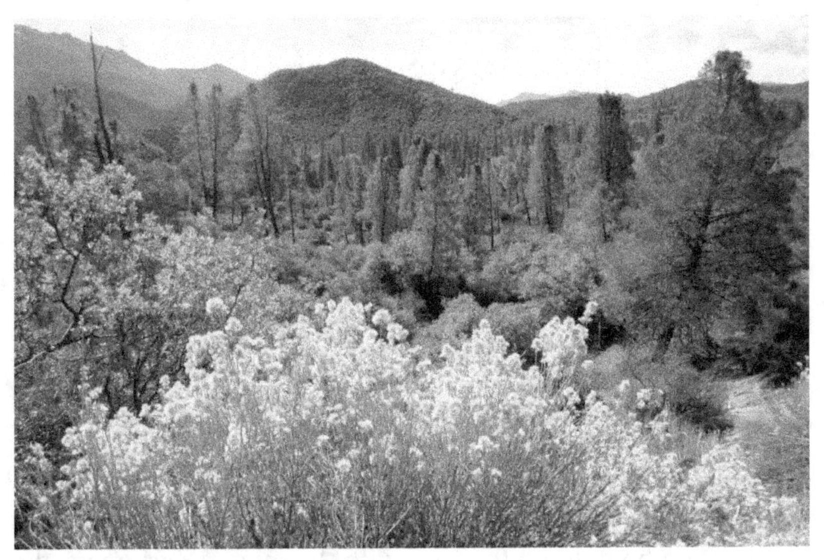

Testimonials

Since I discovered you and The Code, I think: I really found the Truth and Love that I have looked for since my birthday (77 years.)
Friendly
Jean-Pierre

Olga N. Borisenko

I feel privileged to have had an opportunity to read this book. It opens your mind to unknown possibilities, which one would be willing to test with a leap of faith. This book is not one time help; it's a life-changing journey. It's easy to read and understand, though your mind might be skeptical here and there, and in this case, you have to try it out to see the results.

olya.n.borisenko@gmail.com

Eva Garcia

After reading *The lion Moves Alone* by Yuri Spilny two years ago, I was convinced I stumbled upon an exceptional author who can explain difficult concepts and has real authority in what he is sharing. *The Code of Life Communications and System of Health* is a different book because it requires a leap of faith in *The Code* and a willingness to test it and use it. I have been using *The Code* with good results since I first read the book. I re-read the book's parts I did not understand because I saw I was given a powerful help on my spiritual path.

It is not a book to understand with the mind. Yuri opens the world of power: the world of the energy we call Love and beyond. As The Code of Life demonstrates it, love is not an abstract concept but powerful energy we can use to elevate ourselves, achieve better health and relationship with ourselves and others, and have a fulfilled life. I am grateful for the wisdom of the author and his willingness to share it with people.

Eva Garcia
eva@capagencialiteraria.com

Hello,
I am Maher. I met Master Yuri about one year ago. At that time, I had a terrible cold. Because of God and The Code of Life (Master Yuri explained how to use it), in just a few days, I was well.
My father had a health problem for five years: it was difficult for him to move his hands. Master Yuri explained to me how my father could use The Code of Life. It is because of God and The Code of Life that my father is now feeling well. The Code is a real Magician.

Thank God.
And thank you, Master Yuri

Maher's telephone in Egypt +2-0127-638-0902

<u>Explanation</u>

In reality, Maher's father (75) had tremor. *The Code* suggested placing his hands on *The Code* for three to four minutes, four times a day, for about two weeks. I wanted to see how well it would work without charging *The Code*. The man was 97% well in about one week. *The Code* advised to stop this procedure for about thirty days because *The Code,* together with the immune system, was healing the man to a 100% without laying hands on top of it but keeping it somewhere in the house (or in another town☺

Hamada Jamal

Many thanks to my friend Yuri who helped me with the difficult problem I had with my stomach. No doctor could not help me. Mr. Yuri explained to me the reason behind the problem with my stomach. It was some harmful bacteria. The stomach did not digest food properly, I had too much gas, breathing was difficult, and I had a burning sensation in the stomach's pit. Yuri made for me a unique Code. I have used it for two weeks. During this time, the problems were gone one by one. Now I am fine, and I am very grateful to Mr. Yuri. Signed by Hamada Jamal December 22, 2019

Hamada Jamal made his request in January 2019. At that time, I just discovered *The Code of Life* and was researching it. I have created for Hamada Digital Code specific to his problems. Later, I used *The Code of Life* exclusively, as it happened to be the most powerful universal Code.

The Code of Life: **The new powerful method to help your Life.**

When first reading this book, you may not agree with all the author's sentiments, as some of them are very difficult to believe. However, it is essential to look past these and concentrate on the excellent method unveiled!

The first-time reader needs to concentrate on the method; some of the conclusions will make sense later. *The Code* is a truly powerful method for improving one's life, becoming your best teacher and realizing freedom!

I must confess that I have not used *The Code* for physical healing. The first time I filed a request had to do with finding a job. I had been unemployed for about a year, and due to family circumstances, I was not actively seeking employment. As with taking vitamins, I did not do it every day, but I did make a point to feel it when I did. All in all, I would say that I filed the request a total of 20-25 times. One day, out of the blue, I received a call from an acquaintance who begged me to take a job that was not yet posted, but I was the first choice, and would I please take it, which I did!

I was going through a lot of drama in moving out of an apartment, and ex-roommates were spouting such crazy nonsense that it made my head spin. While driving and running through a conversation I had just had with an "ex," I was fuming and getting overwhelmed by negative emotions that had nothing to do with what I could control. In the spur of the moment, I created a request to transform the negative feelings into positive ones. By the time I finished filing the request, I was already feeling a lot better, and now when I think about the situation, it brings up no negative emotions!

The *Code of Life* is a powerful method that will help alter your Life by allowing you to understand and participate in your body's inner workings and mind.

Try it with an open mind and see how far you can get by transforming your darkness into a higher energy level!

Katya K. Long Island, NY

Kat.khell@gmail.com

Daniel S.

The Code of Life Communications and System of Health truly helps one acquire belief in and knowledge of oneself, understand the state of affairs inside and around us, and how all of this can assist in healing oneself first mentally and morally, consequently, physically. Truly amazing.

Szabo Daniel danielszabo@deloittece.com

Ema S.

Hi Yuri,

I hope you are well.

I just wanted to tell you I noticed while doing the Code as you suggested for my thyroid. My taste in food has changed, and for the first time in a long time, there seems to be no hold on me with food. Considering all the techniques I have tried and slimming down products, I think it is amazing.

But the most significant key your book has given me is that you have to charge with emotion, which gives the whole process a great boost.

Thank you so much for all your help.

Wishing you a great day.

Ema

 I have been making a request for my stomach acidity and have only changed some words from the last request you gave me.

Being in a state of love, oh love, I request thy infinite, power to charge my Code of Life with the full strength of thy energy to destroy virus in my bile, rightly orient genes of my bile, as well as to restore my bile acidity.

I saw the difference with my stomach within a few days………………..it felt lighter, I have also been eating more vegetables and generally being more careful with what I eat, but it has never been so easy doing so. Thank you so much for that.
I also asked the code if I could make one more request, and that was about my marriage, and I got the go-ahead, which has been working well for me too……………
How can I ever thank you for discovering something so simple yet so amazing!!!!
Ema

Anda Maric (see reviews on Amazon.com)

I love Yuri's writing. It's easy to read yet deep and makes one think. It reminded me that I always knew that many things he talks about were true, even no one confirmed. This exciting book takes you on a journey that you wish lasts and lasts! I love it!

Maher and Nada. Pain in the arms and the back

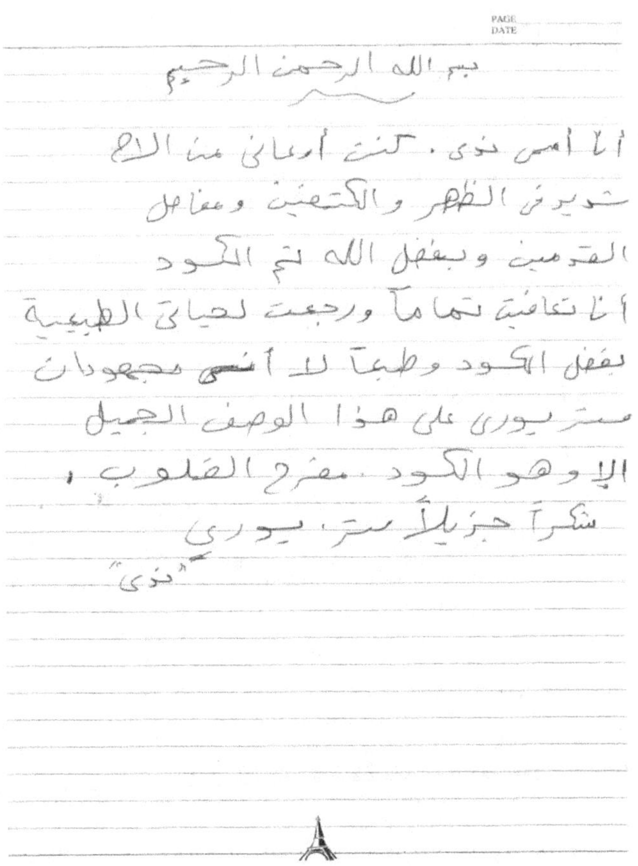

"My name is Nada

I was suffering from back and shoulder pain (For almost three years, doctors and medicine did not help.) Thanks to our Lord and then The Code of Life, I recovered from the pain. I will not forget the effort of Mister Yuri. Thank you so much."

أنا ماهر كنت أعاني من الألم شديدة
في مفصل الكوع الايسر والكتف
وأيضا الآم شديدة في أسفل الظهر العظامية
وبفضل الله ثم "الكود" عن طريق
مستر يوري وتعليماته أنا أحسن
كثير من الأول ونسبة تحسن وصلت من
٧٠ الى ٨٠ ٪ للأفضل الحمد لله ثم الكود .
الكود هو علاج فعال يعمل على
ارسال (الطاقة) الإيجابيه للإنسان
بصورة واضحة وطبيعا كل الشكر
إلى مستر يوري هو صاحب الفضل
في ذلك عن طريق الكود . "ماهر"

"I'm Maher.

I was suffering from pain in the left shoulder (elbow) and pain in the lower back. And after Mister Yuri instructions, I used The Code of Life and have improved by 80%, thank

God. The Code is actually a nice thing to give Positive energy to humans. Thank you, Mister Yuri, for helping me."

Maher and Nada both were holding hands on top of *The Code*. I determined the timing and the number of days for each of them.

Holding Hands on Top of *The Code* works faster for young people. When an older person has 100% Intel-Star energy and higher, there is no difference in the procedure's timing than a young person's.

A letter from Roxie
December 2, 2021

Dear Yuri,

I typed up my journey so far.
After reading A Lion Moves Alone, which was left in the house I am renting, I looked for more of your books as the simplicity of the message was something I had been looking for years. As I was searching, I stumbled upon your email address and messaged to get my Intel-Star level right away. Then I received The Code of Life Communications and Systems of Health and began reading it. I messaged you about my health issues and it took me a few days to figure out how to proceed using specific instructions from you. As I was doing some of the cleansing work, I could feel immediate changes in my body.

Now I use no toothpaste or rinsing with water, only occasional floss for my teeth. I canceled all appointments for dental work, cleanings, and a physical.

I had shoulder tension, which you said was caused by bacteria. You had me put my hands on The Code 4 times a day for 6 minutes for six days, and it disappeared. I had low back pain on the right side for months, if not years. You told me it is Protozoa and bacteria in the ascending colon, which is more common after removing the appendices (mine has not been yet), and The Code instantly destroyed the pathogens. And, of course, I no longer have that. I am very grateful.

For digestive issues, I am on day 4 of 6 of a constipation protocol you gave me. At this point, you switched me over to one copy of The Code of Horus.
Being in the state of Love, oh Love! I request thy infinite energy to charge my Code of Horus to normalize my stomach acid to 3.5. Thank you, thank you, thank you... continue charging for 30 seconds. Today, I went from abnormal stool before and to a normal stool after my first request of the day. It only took less than four days!

I was quite surprised by the food suggestions. I had always thought I was a meat-eater, but I quickly threw out that idea as I realized how easily we adopt the beliefs of those around us and never question them.

The last issue is what looks like 3-degree burns, a patch under my nose, one between my breasts, and one on my right big toe, which turned black and is still black. I was instructed to start working on that after the constipation was corrected.

Thank you for your guidance and love!
With much love,
Roxie

Dear Roxie, as you have your Intel-Star energy level above 80%, use the Intense Healing Mode (it is attached). *Being in the state of Peace, oh, Infinite intelligence, I request thy boundless force to charge my Code of Horus with the full strength of thy energy to destroy all causes inhibiting the health of my skin under my nose, between my breasts, and on my right big toe, and restore my skin.* The pause between procedures should be 30 minutes. You do not need to charge *The Code* for 30 seconds. Please, read the attached. Yuri

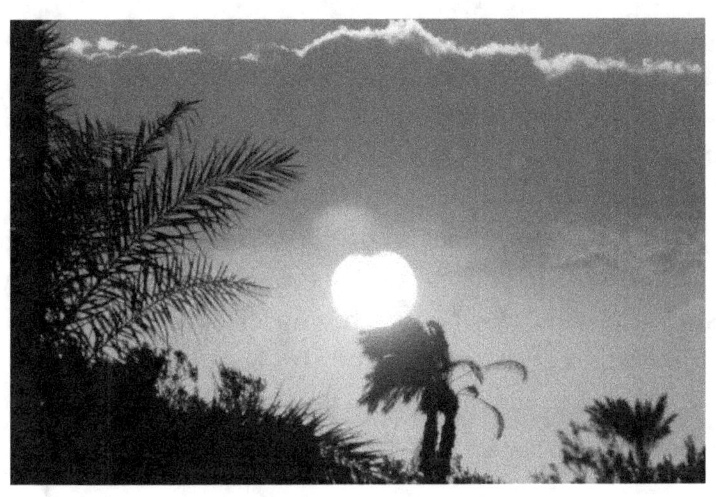

Diagnose and Cure

The System of Health and Healing

The System of Health uses the high-intensity frequency of the high energy level to heal and restore the body and brain.

When the Intel-Star energy level is between 40% and 80%, the System employs The Code of Life and uses its energy as additional help to whatever energy we already have to heal and restore.

The System of Health uses the high-intensity frequency of the high energy level to heal and restore the body and brain.

When the Intel-Star energy level is between 40% and 80%, the System employs The Code of Life. It uses its energy as additional help to heal and restore whatever energy we already have.

We know that in the computer, a system restore point is a backup copy of important Windows operating system (OS) files and settings that can be used to recover the system to an earlier point in the event of system failure or instability.

As our biocomputer keeps the memory of our state of health at our life's every instant, with this system, you could use the restoration of your organs, systems, processes, body, and brain to the state of health of whatever past year you choose. The best date is your birthday because at that time everything is perfect with your body and brain. However, it is important to underline that it should be the health-only Restore point because you do not want to lose things you need to remember.

I request my Biocomputer to establish my Health-only Restore point at my birth on January 2, 1997 and restore my body and brain to the perfection of that state's health.

Even if you have some congenital disabilities, you can restore them to perfect health. To accomplish it, you must find out when the congenital disability happened in the womb or in the process of giving birth, and set your health-only Restore point a few minutes before that time. It can be done with the SP.

Request – the instruction for the biocomputer must be formulated precisely. You may also add a month, a day, or even an hour, but make sure your health is perfect on the chosen date, as you will restore your body and brain's health to the state it was at your restore point.

To use the "Restore" feature, you must have a 180% Intel-Star energy level or higher. You must use the SP to choose the right Restore Point. Check every part of it with the SP.

It is a powerful healing method; however, it requires the utmost confidence and a couple of years of working with The

Code. It also requires extreme accuracy when formulating a request for a Restore point.

When the Intel-Star energy level is between 80% and 150%, the System employs _The Code of Horus_ and uses its 10 to the 6000 power frequency at 300% energy added to what we already have to heal and restore. When _The Code of Horus_ is charged like we charge _The Code of Life_, its energy rises to 700% with 10 to the 100.000 power frequency. I was never advised to charge it because its energy and frequency in a free state were always enough to do the job. For you, it may be different.

To use "Restore" feature, you must have a 180% Intel-Star energy level or higher. You must use the SP to chose the right Restore Point. Check every part of it with the SP.

It is a powerful healing method; however, it also requires an utmost confidence and a couple years of working with The Code. It also requires an extreme acuracy when formulating a request for Restore point.

> Eventually, you would be led to the simplest universal method, "Laying Hands." Depending on your state of health, age, Intel-Star energy level, other features, and the nature of the disease, you will place your hands on The Code several times a day for several minutes each time. The numbers can be determined only with the SP. As you do not yet master the SP, you may request assistance at yuri@bookstoenjoy.com.

You could aid laying hands mode with a simple request without going into details:

Being in the state of peace, Oh Infinite intelligence, I request you destroy all cases inhibiting my liver and restore my liver to the state of perfect health. To use this method, your energy level must be 175%
While keeping your hands on The Code, be completely relaxed, having no thoughts, just watching your mind.

Using the energy of the Infinite Intelligence

At birth, we are given everything necessary to create and live a life of happiness and success. Our Intel-Star (*soul*) has a 100% energy level with a frequency of 10 to the 56 power, which is the energy and frequency of Love. It is necessary for people to become their best and only teachers. However, from day one, we are introduced to negativity, lies, and deception by self-appointed teachers and often by parents who know no love. We must strive to become our best and only teachers, using our energy resource and, when necessary, assisting it with the energy of The code of Life or Horus. Nevertheless, it may not be enough to cure some health issues. Then, start using the powerful energy of Infinite Intelligence as your last resource. This resource has a very high level of energy and frequency that cannot be fathomed. Also, its frequency has no upper limit.

Being in the state of peace, oh, Infinite intelligence, I request you to use your powerful energy to destroy all causes inhibiting my eyes including fungus, Viruses, Protozoa, and bacteria, and through it all out. Eradicate astigmatism, and restore regeneration processes in my eyes and restore my eyes to perfection of health.

It is recommended Using the above in the Intense Healing method, repeating the affirmation every thirty minutes.

When the Intel-Star energy level is between 80% and 150%, the System employs *The Code of Horus* and uses its 10 to the 6000 power frequency at 300% energy added to what we already have to heal and restore. When *The Code of Horus* is charged like we charge *The Code of Life*, its energy rises to 700% with 10 to the 100.000 power frequency. I was never advised to charge it because its energy and frequency in a free state were always enough to do the job. For you it may be different.

When the Intel-Star energy level is between 150% and 175%, the System employs *The Code of Horus+*; it cannot be charged because, in its free state, it has more than enough power to do the job. In its free state, it has a 10.000% energy level and 10 to the 10 million power frequency.

When the Intel-Star energy level is above 175%, the System employs no *Code* but uses the energy of Love.

As you can notice, the higher our energy level, the more powerful *Code* we are offered. We gradually come to the point when no Code is needed, and Love or Infinite Intelligence guides us. I did not find out why it is not just *Infinite Intelligence,* as Love is a part of it. Maybe you will figure it out.

The System of Health encourages us to raise our Intel-Star energy level.

Information in this chapter is written for people with 52% to 80% Intel-Star energy levels. When your energy is above 80%, adjust it accordingly, like using *The Code of Horus* and destroying the causes instead of particular reasons: pathogens, deposits, pesticides, etc. However, it may be necessary to add specific reasons for the restoration and orientation of genes in some cases.

When making inquiries and diagnoses, it is necessary to start your question as:

I request the Infinite Intelligence to let me know if I should use the power of Love or the boundless force of Infinite Intelligence etc.

Unlike the destruction of pathogens, deposits in blood vessels, restoration of genomes, etc., you may destroy the causes of the ailment without going into detail.

Your energy level must be 80% and higher to use this method.

Being in the state of love, oh love, I request you destroy all causes inhibiting my eyes ,restore regeneration processes to perfection, and restore my eyes to perfection of health.

It is used mostly with the Intense Healing Mode.

Also, persons with an 80% Intel-Star energy and higher should use one page with the image of Horus printed on both sides of the page instead of *The Code of Life (*keep it in the fridge).

When your Intel-Star energy level is 175%, you will heal any disease with a request programming your Biocomputer. *The Code* is not needed. A 175% energy level is sufficient to eliminate the causes of the disease, restore and rightly orient genes, and restore organs, systems, processes, tissue, bones, nerves, and dissolve deposits in blood vessels.

Being in the state of Love, I request you to destroy all causes inhibiting my Thalamus and Inter-thalamic adhesion and restore my Thalamus and Inter-thalamic adhesion to perfection of health.

Being in the state of Love, I request you to destroy all causes inhibiting my body and brain, remove, restore regeneration processes to perfection, and restore my body and brain to perfection of health.

It may sound too simple, and it is: the procedure is simplicity itself. At 175% of Intel-Star's energy level, we use our innate ability to restore health without using *The Code (s)*. Raise your Intel-Star's energy level and experience this beautiful state.

At a 175% energy level, our Biocomputer is freed from nearly all impediments (medical science, cultural rigmarole, teachers, teachings, and other human-created nonsense) and can perform its natural functions. One of these functions is focusing Intel-Star energy provided by its core on the causes of the disease, destroying these causes, thus, eliminating the disease. Another – is performing accurate diagnoses. Yet, another – receiving precise information to our inquiries, and so forth.

From experience, I found that there may be a time when no request is necessary, letting the body and brain take care of the issue. In this case, I found, our biocomputer connects to Infinite intelligence and uses the energy of the Intel-Star's core to accomplish what is necessary. No interference is needed on our part. Aways consult your SP or use The Master of Simplicity method. Your energy level must be close to

200% for your biocomputer to employ this method without your help.

Below 175% Intel-Star energy level, our Biocomputer is still plagued with some obstructions and cannot efficiently focus Intel-Star energy to restore what needs to be restored. In this case, we have to use additional help: the energy of *The Code of Life, The Code of Horus,* or *The Code of Horus +.*

Nothing in the universe comes close to the human body and brain's beauty and organization. Just look at the cells secreting renin or Glomerulus in the renal tissue. A renal glomerulus filter blood. It is made of narrow arteries and resembles a ball of tangled yarn. It is only 0.2 mm. in diameter, and it does such an incredible job. I cannot stop wondering about this miracle called the Human body.

This is a new discovery. I tested it many times: it works fine. <u>We must add to every request</u> *a request to restore regeneration process to perfection for a particular organ, system and process*:

Being in the state of peace, oh, Infinite Intelligence, I request you to destroy all causes inhibiting my eyes; and in my eyes, restore regeneration processes and restore my eyes to perfection of health.

When charged, the Code's energy rises to 200% with 10 to the *6000 power frequency*. This incredible benevolent power enables *The Code's* limitless capabilities. With *The Code,* you will eradicate all that obstructs Life and restore all that needs to be restored for the body to thrive and life to flourish.

Even without being charged, *The Code* generates 100% energy with a frequency of ten to the 56 power, which is powerful enough to eliminate arthritis or tremor when hands are laid on *The Code* for a few minutes several times a day.

When we request information related to the body and mind, answers are provided by our Biocomputer, the brain that has complete knowledge of the body. When we file a healing request, our Biocomputer focuses our energy aided by the energy of *The Code* on the target and, fulfills our request. External information about the human world, relationships, business, finances, Nature, and the Universe we are receiving from the *Infinite Intelligence.* Nevertheless, in many instances, we use *the boundless force of the Infinite Intelligence* for healing. Consult *The Code.*

The Code of Life is a breakthrough in diagnoses and cures. With it you will diagnose and heal every disease, from the common cold to cancer. With *The Code,* you can do every test from Blood P.H. to heart tissue P.H., Cholesterol, PSA, Hormones, Blood sugar, stones in kidneys and bladder, and dissolve the stones. You will dissolve deposits in arteries and veins, restore the heart and other organs, restore and improve sexual health, and monitor healing progress.

You do not need to be a subject of medical science's mistakes and often -- ignorance. You do not need to poison your body with medicines' side effects. Become your best and only doctor. Accurately diagnose yourself, and when treatment is necessary, do it with beneficial high-frequency energy incomparably more efficiently than doctors and medicines.

According to the research, we get all our physical energy from food. The food must have 95% energy and higher to provide energy. Food with lower than 95% energy level does not provide energy but is converted to fat (sugar 75%, meat 34%, fish 17%, all processed food 23%).

There is an energoinformational connection between our biocomputer and an outer field of Intel-Star. The biocomputer sends to Intel-Star information about the state of our brain-body system and personality, enabling us to "read" this information about any person in the way of inquiries/energy levels.

For example, when we ask, "How greedy is David on the scale of 100%?" We receive a reply from David's Intel-Star's outer field.

However, when we ask, "How healthy is my liver on a zero to 100% scale?" We receive a reply from our biocomputer that knows all about our body and brain.

A reply from the Infinite Intelligence we receive via several receptors in the brain. You may not differentiate between the Infinite Intelligence and the infinite field of knowledge because it is <u>only</u> the all-inclusive Infinite Intelligence. Your Intel-Star energy level must be above 120% to receive information exclusively from the Infinite intelligence <u>about everything</u>, including the body and brain. The receptors in the brain become active at 120% when they are freed from all garbage that was clogging them.

It is also Oneness, as we are immersed in the Infinite Intelligence like fish in water, which means we are forever in the state of Oneness. However, our Intel-Star energy level must be at least 120% to become conscious of it. It must be 175% to experience it.

A human body and brain need little meat (no red meat) and very little fish. Because it clogs the system and takes much energy to process and eliminate. There are always exceptions. Chicken soup with brown rice, carrots, and onion has an energy of 150% and is good to have two-three times a week.

But widely advertised Fish Oil has nothing that the body could use. It is harmful to the liver.

Term Calorie is useless and misleading; it has deficient (below52%) energy level.

"Calorie, a unit of energy or heat ***variously defined***?). The calorie was originally defined as the amount of heat required at a pressure of 1 standard atmosphere to raise the temperature of 1 gram of water 1° Celsius."

It is impossible to understand calory because it is an artificial concept. It fails to define energy. Because medical science is incapable of measuring the energy level and frequency of the foodstuff, it created calory. It is the same medical ignorance as bloodletting used for centuries by the "doctors" on every occasion. Unfortunately, a common medical stupidity found its way into our century because most doctors remain talentless, ignorant, low energy people.

The food provides the body with a lower (comparing Intel-Star's) energy and frequency. The body converts any food with energy below 95% to fat. Examples are, including "natural," drinks 31%; Coca-Cola 61%.

The body needs eggs, cheese, milk, honey, some grains, a small amount of vegetables, carrots, cabbage, berries, nuts, and much fruits. Fruits, not vegetables, are the prime builders of the body. As to the vegetables, only a few of them are useful. Leafy vegetables are all useless; tomatoes, potatoes, and so forth must be cooked; check it out with *The Code.*

The Code of Life Communications and System of Health is truly a future of medicine when people will diagnose and heal themselves.

With *The Code* we can check every decision related to business, finances, relationships, employees, and any person in the world, dead or alive. We could evaluate people's kindness, honesty, sincerity, selfishness, greed, etc.

In 1989, before establishing *USSR Film Service Corp.* representing Soviet Film Industry in Hollywood, I met a Russian man named Dan. He was a young, energetic, and friendly person. His home was in San Francisco, and he lived in my Santa Monica apartment on 23-d Street. When the company was established, I made Dan my partner. I knew nothing about the energy levels. Dan and I divided our responsibilities: he took care of the Russian end, and I was making deals in Hollywood.

In several years, *USSR Film Service Corp.* facilitated many Russian-American co-productions. In the end, I found out Dan was making deals in Russia behind my back. Before I let Dan go, we signed an agreement listing the projects that Dan and I developed in the past several years. Soon I learned Dan was secretly doing our projects in Russia. I learned Dan's energy level was below 12% when I discovered The Code.

You have the all-powerful *Code of Life.* Use it and partner with persons who have 80% and above energy levels. It is also crucial in marriage. The difference between the <u>man and the woman's</u> energy levels must be less than 12%. There must be a spiritual, physical, and mental affinity.

The Code is available to transgender people as their average Intel-Star energy level is around 80%, eliminating speculation and prejudges about transgender people. Having their energy level higher than an average American or Russian person, transgender folks are more loving and, in general, are in many ways better than many so-called "normal" people.

With *The Code of Life,* we can determine if certain information or a book is helpful without opening it, even without having it. There is no end to the wonders of this system. With *The Code of Life,* in the valley two miles away from my land, I discovered 9.5 billion barrels of oil. *The Code* makes anyone capable of uncovering secrets. To begin with, we are primarily interested in accurate diagnosis, cure, and staying healthy.

The higher your energy level, the more efficient the healing process and the more accurate replies you get to queries.

"When it comes to the diagnosis, we are still in shadows," said my friend Marry Erickson MD. Every doctor knows it. With *The Code of Life,* we can accurately diagnose every organ and identify the cause of every disease. We receive and verify this information accurately, leaving contemporary medicine in the stone age.

My other friend's daughter is a heavy smoker. I found that 13% of her left lung was cancerous (I should not have made this diagnosis, a rule I discovered later). When I mentioned it to the mother (also a doctor), she was upset not because of cancer but because she believed in nothing but the conventional tests. Yet, with *The Code,* we learn out of 100 patients with less than 20% of lung cancer, CAT Scan misses cancer in about 70 cases.

During our Life, we collect and store a lot of garbage in our mental/physical system. When I began using *The Code,* I discovered many health issues to attend to. When I diagnosed the heart, P.H. of the ventricles, atriums, and apex cordis was between 5.5 and 6.6, which resulted in the muscles' effectiveness ratio between 45% and 60% (instead of 100%.) The efficiency ratio demonstrates the effectiveness of the organ's performance. Two lung veins have been clogged with deposits. My aorta was at 60%. In about two months, I normalized all issues.

I traced pathogens when they invaded my heart and other organs and found out most of it had happened during surgery when heavy anesthetics compromised the body's defense. I also learned that my proximity to some people with a low energy level negatively affects my health. Medical science's sluggishness prevents doctors' understanding of the simple fact: a person with a low Intel-Star energy level could inhance illness in people around him. Considering the energy-deficient state of US medicine, with 95% of doctors' energy levels below 52%, it is no wonder.

A cold usually would take me from ten days to two weeks to recuperate. With *The Code of Life,* the cold was gone by the second day's morning and never returned. In Egypt, I helped several people to eliminate the flu in just two days.

A tissue P.H. test of the liver and other organs is expensive and rarely done. These tests are often critical. With *The Code of Life,* we can perform every test, including tissue P.H., PSA, good, bad, and total cholesterol, the presence of cancer, and the effectiveness ratio of every organ, system, process, and its components. There is no need for scans, X-rays, or any equipment. We can perform hormonal analyses, ventilation, blood pressure, temperature, deposits in the arteries and veins, stones in the liver, bladder, and other organs, and dissolve the deposits and stones exclusively with *The Code of Life.* We candetermine the causes of the issues and cure ourselves of any condition.

I repeat this statement throughout the book: <u>healing can be performed without the Star Pendulum (The S.P.)</u>. Still, I recommend mastering the S.P. and becoming the Master of Simplicity. It would enable you to perform tests, do diagnoses, calculate the number of charges, and do other things necessary to be your best and only doctor.

Our body makes almost all the necessary nutrients. What it does not make, it absorbs from food. With *The Code of Life,* we can restore the production of the nutrients often inhibited by the unnecessary consumption of supplements and choose what is necessary. In one month, I restored the nutrient production and discarded 14 bottles of supplements – all I had. How long would it take us to do with a doctor or nutritionists

I had a high B.P. for decades. As I cleaned and restored the body and brain, my B.P. went down to one hundred. *The Code* advised me it was normal and that it would take some time for the body to adjust and for B.P. to normalize. Almost two years later, as I add new information to the book, my B.P. is 110/69.

At 80, after stomach surgery, my life resource was 14 months. At that time, I discovered *The Code of Life* and healed the body and brain, raising the resource to twenty-three years.

When you fine-tune *The Code of Life*, the S.P., and your Biocomputer (the brain), you will be able to check the accuracy of every statement in this book and be convinced of The Code of Life's precision.

After discovering *The Code,* we made many a hundred tests proving the effectiveness of the system's many aspects.

I am convinced it is my purpose to make this gift of Life available to all people. So that all may enjoy a life of health, free of doctors and medications, and food and water free of contaminants.

It is apparent healing any disease, from the common cold to cancer, could be executed by merely resting hands on *The Code* for a specific time. The length, the number of repetitions, and the days can be determined depending on the nature of the disease, age, and Intel-Star energy level.

In the beginning, use regular healing methods discussed in this chapter. You will be guided as of when to start using the "Laying your hands upon *The Code*" method.

Thus, we now have powerful healing means that anyone can use without doctors, medicine, and equipment. It requires one page of *The Code* printed on each side of the page and brief instructions.

You may be interested in learning how many reasons are causing, for example, the malfunction of your right kidney. Do not be surprised if the number of causes may be as high as nine or more.

For people with Intel-Star energy levels of 80% and up, start your request with something like this:

Being in the state of Peace, Oh, Infinite Intelligence, I request you to destroy all causes inhibiting my right kidney, restore it, etc. You are using Infinite Intelligence's power, not Love's power.

In most cases, destroying the causes would enable healing without going into the details, like identifying and eliminating pathogens, deposits, etc. However, it may be necessary to destroy a particular pathogen or dissolve a deposit of calcium, fat, and salt along with the destruction of the causes. Feel free to experiment and compare results.

People with Intel-Star lower than 80% need to identify and eliminate every cause, like a particular pathogen, deposit in the vessels, etc. It is all individual

Once, before I learned about the Destruction of the causes, I felt discomfort in the body's right side above the hip after eating fish. Using the Atlas of the Human Body, I looked for pathogens in the duodenum. When the presence of the pathogens was confirmed, I destroyed them:

Being in the state of Love, Oh Love, I request you to destroy protozoa, fungus, and worms in my duodenum and throw this garbage out of my body. Thank you! Thank you!, Thank you!

Again, I checked the duodenum for pathogens; there were none. The discomfort also was gone. Truly amazing! When something like this happens, it is good to check out other organs. In my case, the intruders made their way into the liver and pancreas.

Your request must be precise as your Biocomputer uses it to focus your and *The Code's* energy on the target detailed in the request. Check your request for accuracy before and after you file it. Ask if it is 100% correct. If it is not, check out every part of the request and correct it accordingly. Ensure whether you need to use the power of Love or *Infinite Intelligence.* Soon, you will notice, it is energy of Love that is usually used to destroy pathogens.

Check it for accuracy when the same request is used for a long time because some request details could have changed during the healing process. For example, in Ken's request to restore the urinary tract, it was no longer necessary to destroy fungus, viruses, and bacteria after filing it for two days.

<u>To ensure healing is maximum effective, healing requests must be formulated precisely. With the request, biocomputer will focus your plus *The Code's* energy on the target as if you aim at it with a rifle. You do not need to name particular bacteria. You must name the pathogen's type (bacteria, protozoa, worms, viruses, or fungus) and pinpoint the pathogen's location.</u>

You will find the details in the Intense Healing Mode of the Advanced Healing Method. You may find it is no longer necessary to place your hands on *The Code*.

Medical science overall utilizes 50% and lower energy levels. It is why medical science is often ineffective: it works on low-level energy with the corresponding low frequency. It is low because many US doctors have average energy levels below 52%. These doctors should not be allowed to practice, as they could harm their patients.

The Code of Life utilizes high frequency energy and is incomparably more efficient at diagnosing and healing than any medicine. Also, *The Code* does not need money and cannot be corrupted☺ It enables everyone to heal himself and discard medications along with side effects.

Medical science does not recognize the principal role of energy in healing. It is understandable as science cannot register frequencies above ten to the thirty-five power, but *The Code* can. Conventional science is always lagging behind discoveries that have to fight their way to acceptance. The pharmaceutical industry does not want people to know they are self-sufficient and can heal themselves without drugs.

Medical science does not see viruses, protozoa, fungi, worms, and bacteria as the cause of the disease. Not having the right knowledge, it is treating illness with chemicals. It has been conditioned by the pharmaceutical industry to turn away from any other way of healing, no matter how beneficial. It goes as far as depriving doctors of their licenses when they try to use effective alternative methods. Another reason is that 87% of doctors globally have low energy and an average IQ of 81, so their minds could hardly be open to the knowledge they did not receive in college.

In over six years of diagnosing and healing with *The Code,* I found it, with rare exceptions, pathogens are only the cause of the disease in addition to genetic damage, changes in molecular structure, and deposits of calcium, cholesterol, fat, and salt. Even in schizophrenia, pathogens are the main cause of illness. For example, in leg cramps, the cause is bacteria, protozoa, and fungus in the muscles of the legs that are easily eliminated with the beneficial high-frequency energy of *The Code.* Of course, the initial cause may be something like inheritance, severe cold, or a shock. But the real and treatable causes are pathogens that damage tissue and bones, disrupt systems and processes, and disorient and damage genes and neurons.

The Code's healing ability is another issue. How does it destroy pathogens, pesticides, and chemicals in people, foods, and water, leaving all that is useful and valuable intact? How does *The Code* restore tissue, processes, systems, and organs? It is possible that when *The Code* eliminates the culprit, our immune system does the rest of the healing. The mechanics of the healing process need to be researched. Our experience confirms that we quickly and effectively perform healing with *The Code.*

The Code's energy is benevolent, which means it creates and supports all that helps advance life; it destroys all that inhibits life. We do not yet learn mechanics, but every case of healing proves this incredible ability of *The Code.*

Unless they stop violating the laws of nature and stop their harmful activity, people with low energy levels will keep harming others and destroying themselves with their long-wave, low-frequency energy. The higher the frequency, the more efficient the energy at performing positive tasks and doing good. The energy of an unimaginable high frequency is incomprehensibly intelligent.

Our humanity and the universe are likely to be "an experiment" made by the Infinite Intelligence "to see" if its unimaginable high frequency is also possible in the physical universe and a human being. It may look like an idea of socialism that was corrupted in the case of the USSR because of the masses' low 39% Intel-Star energy level (in 1937) and corresponding 86 IQ. Although much less brutal than in the recent times of the Catholic inquisition (with the masses' 19% overall Intel-Star energy level) led by the half-humans called the popes (9% overall energy level), corruption is still taking place today in humanity's growth on its way to perfection. Today, the overall Intel-Star energy level of our humanity is 39%. With such a low energy level, it cannot elect the high energy level leaders but chooses Biden, Trudeau, Macron, and other human trash.

Nevertheless, human evolution is always upwards, despite temporary setbacks caused by religious ignorance bordering on stupidity and devastating wars like WWI and WWII. Xi Jumping, Maduro, Al Sisi, and Donald Trump indicate a positive trend in humanity's inner growth.

Destruction of what is inhibiting life and restoring and preserving life is *The Code's* purpose with its ever-higher frequency with no known upper limit. An average person cannot generate energy with a frequency higher than ten to the 56 power we call True Love. When it is charged, *The Code* provided in this book generates a frequency of 10 to the 6000 power, which, when it is focused on the target, is capable of changing the molecular structure of tissue, repairing and orienting genes in the right direction, reconnecting neurons, and do many other astonishing things. Every healing performed with *The Code of Life* supports this statement.

Whether medical science agrees, *The Code of Life* does incredible things. The proof is that we get well without doctors, medicines, and equipment with *The Code of Life* – medicine of the future. Like anything utterly novel, *The Code's* System of Health will continue to experience criticism, even attacks, until the old kicks the bucket.

Before reading further, look through the Atlas of the human body and be amazed at the excellent machine our body is, then comprehend our Biocomputer, the brain, manages this beautiful system. We are in charge of this wonder.

When diagnosing a particular organ or system, looking at the related picture in the Atlas is instrumental.

Before making diagnoses, raise your energy level as suggested in the *Key Points* in the sub-chapter *Elevating energy level*. Diagnoses are made with the SP or Simplicity method.

It is also wise to perform your diagnosis when diagnosed with a particular disease. The results may surprise you.

To get started, make a list of the body systems. You would find it in an atlas or on the Web. I prefer the atlas. It is another wonder how moving the SP over the picture of the liver, we are scanning our liver instantly and confirming the presence of pathogens in our liver and if there are disoriented or damaged genes or some other issues. How is a picture in the atlas connected to the actual liver? A puzzle! Yet, it is firmly connected, and the scanning produces accurate results. Unlike results produced by CT or any other scan, X-Rays, or ultrasound, our scanning provides accurate results. Also, we see when there are disoriented or damaged genes.

Diagnose every system by letting the SP fly horizontally over every name on the list or using the Simplicity method. You may verbalize every name or ask, "Does it have problems, pathogens, or genetic damage?" Do not strain. You may repeat the check several times to ensure nothing is missing. Add to the list the organs you wish to check first. Then, check the Effectiveness Ratio of the systems and organs you added. It will give you a good picture of your state of health. After that, move on to the details.

When we diagnose ourselves or someone else, we first look for bacteria, viruses, worms, fungus, protozoa, hormones, heavy metals, cancer, deposits of salt, fat, cholesterol, and calcium, and for genetic damage, whether IGD (Inherited Genetic Damage) or the one caused by the negativity (shocks) that changed genes orientation or caused damage to genes.

When you have an infection and want to know what kind of pathogen is causing it, you may search the Web for a list of viruses. Look at the list and one by one name every virus while letting the SP fly free along the imaginary horizontal line. When the SP starts changing direction, it is your virus. Check it out again, asking, "Is it what I have, yes or not?"

You must get "Yes" when your choice is correct. You also may use the Simplicity method.

In Egypt, Maher (51% of energy level), my door attendant, visited his family and returned sick with flu. I gave him a simple code to get rid of it but could not explain how to use it. He did not speak English. Then I asked my longtime friend Isaak, who spoke good English, to help. Smiling, he agreed. In a few days, I realized Isaak was avoiding me. When I checked *The Code*, I learned Isaak's minister advised him *The Code* is Black magic. I also knew Isaak was at a 9% energy level, and his minister had 13%. I found a pharmacist (80% of the energy level) who spoke excellent English, and in a couple of days, Maher was well.

Another time in Egypt, I met a man called Petro. He was pleasant person and knowledgeable. We had lovely walks along the Red Sea coastline. In about four months, I flew back to my Sierra Nevada Mountains. A few months passed, and I was rushed to emergency surgery. There was a pain in my side, so severe it was unbearable. Afterward, Doctor Moon, a brilliant 33-year-old surgeon at the Bakersfield Community Hospital, said he was surprised to see me alive with the stomach infection that should have killed me long before being dropped onto his operating table.

Later, I determined that with Dr. Moon doing surgery, I had only a 7% chance of dying; his Intel-Star energy was 88%. If operated by an equally talented surgeon with an energy level of 12% or less, I would have a 65% chance of dying because of the doctor's damaging negative energy and corresponding low IQ, which means a greater chance of making a mistake leading to death.

The Code of Life says in America, about 60% of severe surgery patients die every year because the surgeon and assisting personnel's powerful low-frequency energy increases the chance of dying. When you are scheduled for surgery, check your surgeon's energy level. If it is less than 70%, choose another surgeon.

The average energy level of all doctors in the US is 21%. 26% of these doctors are engaged in some degenerate, harmful activity. The energy level of these doctors is an average of 8%. Avoid these doctors like the plague.

A doctor must have no less than a 155% energy level to provide a sound professional service. The overall percentage of doctors with a 75% energy level and higher is only 5% in the US.

Soon, Petro and I met in Egypt again, and we spent time together. I was 81 and researching *The Code of Life,* which eventually became this book. I was still recuperating from the surgery, and my body was quite weak. I noticed that some of the resolved health issues had to be attended to again. Luckily, I had *The Code of Life* and was determined to find the reasons for my weakness.

In about two months, I suddenly felt nauseous. The following night I could hardly sleep because of the pain in the right side. The symptoms pointed to another stomach infection. Using the Atlas, I located bacteria (Early Satiety, protozoa, and Acetobacter Acety Xilinus) in the Duodenum. A detailed atlas of the human body and the S.P. are the only tools you would ever need in diagnosing any health issue.

The Code advised me to make 13 request charges with 35 minutes intervals (unusually short intervals). These numbers can be determined only with the SP or Simplicity method.

That day I slept five hours, waking every 35 minutes to charge *The Code* and falling back asleep. By seven PM, the pain was gone. I slept two more hours, woke up, and laughed at how smoothly it worked out compared to the previous stomach infection that nearly took me off this earth.

The following realization happened strangely. I have been charging The Code of Life with minor healing requests daily. One morning, I was about to charge *The Code* but was advised it was unnecessary. I had four requests, yet, I could not charge one. I knew there were some health issues, but *The Code* kept telling me all four requests were satisfied. I obeyed and decided to have a break. When *The Code* advises you to interrupt your healing process, always ask if you need to restart it later.

In the evening, I watched a pristine turquoise sky just before the sunset when it hit me, Petro! Instantly, I checked his energy level. It was below 10%. I never felt relaxed with Petro but tried not to pay attention to it.

One reason for my stomach surgery, weakness, and second stomach infection was Petro's destructive low-frequency energy. I had never suspected Petro's energy level was that low. His long waves of low-frequency energy kept making me ill. *The Code* advised me to drop this relationship unless Petro would raise his energy level to above 52%. It was OK to talk over social networks, but no pictures of Petro were allowed. Of course, a bacterium was the prime cause of stomach infection. If Petro's distracting low energy were not aiding it, my immune system would get rid of it.

When we are young and healthy, someone's low energy is hardly damaging. We become more vulnerable when we get older.

The story of Petro was tragic. He was 63 years old when he got cancer. I knew I could help him with *The Code of Life*, but there was one condition: he had to raise his energy level to above 52%, which means to stop his degenerate way of life. He loved my suggestion but never made use of it. He died of a heart attack shortly after surgery.

At a 15% energy level, the long waves will start disorienting genes in the Right Cerebral Hemisphere of the brain and Hypophyses, Cerebellum, Medulla Oblongata, Pons, and Mesencephalon. It would cause genetic disorders, adversely affect the protein function in genes, and inhibit health and natural development. The destructive activity would also inhibit the SOD1 gene that makes a protein that cures DNA damage in neurons.

The longer the low energy level and the low-frequency energy attack, the more damage it does to genes, which may lead to cancer.

Over 83% of all cancer patients in the US have an average energy level of 15% or under. If this 83% is considered 100%, more than 99% of these people will die from cancer. These statistics are forever the same. It does not change because a person with a low energy level must increase it to be cured. That would happen when one drops abnormal, harmful activity, stops violating nature's laws, and cleans the past of negativity. It is something that people with low energy levels reject doing.

They do not want or cannot leave their offensive, harmful, or weird ways of life for various reasons despite the absolute necessity to increase their energy level. When this condition is disregarded, no cure will help. That is how evolution protects humanity from destruction.

It is evolutionary encouragement for people to increase their energy level and eliminate negativity – the major cause of all human problems. If this low energy issue is left unattended, it, like fungus, may destroy a nation. The increasingly high number of citizens with deficient energy destroyed the Roman Empire and Greece.

Harmful/negative activity is anything a person with an energy level above 52% will not do and would not encourage others to do. It is starting a war, being an invader, usurper, fraud, deceitful, doing unnatural things like smoking, drugs, drinking, or anything that puts brakes on progress, natural human activity, development, and procreation. It is anything contrary to the Truth. Every warmonger of the past and present had their energy level below 15% and was killed either in fighting or by cancer:

Genghis Khan cancer, energy 15%
Alexander the Great cancer, energy 9%
Tamerlane cancer, energy 7%
Attila the Hun cancer, energy 9%
Charlemagne cancer, energy 9%
Thutmose III cancer, energy 11%
Asoka the Great, cancer, energy 9%
Truman cancer, energy 8%
Lenin cancer, energy 5%
Stalin cancer, energy 5%
Hitler cancer, energy 4%
And many others

When you diagnose yourself with pathogens and disoriented or damaged genes, creating two separate requests is often more effective: one for destroying pathogens and another for restoring genes. Some of the following examples have pathogens and genes issues in one request. Please, break them into two requests when necessary. However, there are always exclusions; sometimes, creating two separate requests is unnecessary.

Cancer. The main cause of cancer is a low energy level. There may also be other reasons, such as inheritance, emotional disruption, lifestyle, etc.

It is true that cancer is incurable, but only in people refusing to halt their harmful, unnatural activity that is drastically lowering their energy level. Cancer can develop even at a 65% energy level, like lung cancer in a heavy smoker.

An average American has about 65% energy level. Cancer (AIDS-related cancers, any cancer) is rare and curable at that level. When the energy level drops, the chance of having cancer increases. When the energy level drops to 20%, the possibility of cancer increases to 92%. The cancers are incurable until the patient's energy level rises above 60%. There are exceptions to this rule, as you will see further.

In the past, Bill was engaged in some damaging activities. He had a 13% energy level when he got prostate cancer. He decided to use Ozone and Cannabis and nothing of conventional cure to kill cancer. A brave decision, but over six years of this "treatment," cancer spread to some organs and the skeleton. Bill asked for help, and we explained how to raise the energy level. In about three weeks, with our service, Bill increased his energy level to 85% using the *Elevating energy level* technique. Together we destroyed cancer in every part of the body, including skeleton.

Surprisingly, the following medical test showed cancer in the skeleton and other body parts, where *The Code* eliminated it. That was strange because cancer does not return soon when *The Code of Life* eliminates it. We kept checking Bill: there was no cancer anywhere, but again, medical tests registered cancer while *The Code of Life* showed none.

Eventually, we solved the riddle. Bill kept using Ozone. He was sold by an Internet blogger who was more of a "blabber" glorifying ozone, he had been using it for several years. He kept doing insufflations, claiming that he could not go to the bathroom without it. He kept drinking ozonized water and doing ozone saunas.

With *The Code,* we determined Ozone is poison and should not be used by anybody. Indeed, it helps one to the bathroom, but at the same time, it causes 97% of the damage. We found all information about Ozone on the Internet to be wishful thinking. Eventually, we determined why the "cancer" came back after being eliminated.

Ozone is deadly. Opposite to the Ozone users' widespread opinion, Ozone is not transformed into oxygen when it enters the human body. When Ozone is used for about 12 months (this number would be slightly different for different people), it begins to modify healthy cells, so they appear cancerous. These cells are less aggressive than cancerous cells. Unlike cancerous cells, they do not multiply out of control but test carcinogenic. Ozone was also destroying calcium in Bill's skeleton, causing pain and gradually making Bill immobile. Bill did not believe that and kept using Ozone. Eventually, Bill could not walk. One day he fell, fractured his neck, and was transferred to the hospital. Ozone did its deadly job, and Bill died, killed not by cancer but by Ozone.

Alzheimer. Protozoa and worms invading the spinal cord and the Callosum's Torus are the usual causes of Alzheimer's disease. It weakens these brain and spinal cord parts, damaging genes and disrupting the neuron system, creating Alzheimer's.

To cure Alzheimer's disease, you must use the *Intense Healing Mode*, repeating the procedure every 30 minutes throughout the day. At the end of the day, you would be hinted to stop the procedure for this day. Trust yourself. You could also check it with the *Simplicity Method* or the SP. We highly recommend this method which takes a little time to master. To use the Intense Healing Mode, you must have an 80% Intel-Star energy level (see: *Elevating energy level.*)

To cure Alzheimer's with *The Code*, a patient must have at least an 80% Intel-Star energy level. When someone wants to assist in curing Alzheimer's, their energy level must be 95% or higher.

Being in the state of Love, Oh Love, I request thy infinite power to charge my Code of Life with the full strength of thy energy to destroy worms and Protozoa in my Spinal cord and Torus of the Callosum. Wipe all impurities out of my brain and spinal cord, and restore my brain to perfection of health.

Thank you, thank you, and keep charging *The Code* for 30 seconds.

With high frequency energy, you destroy pathogens. The power of *The Code of Life* is at our command to sustain life and destroy whatever inhibits life.

Blood Pressure. I have had a high BP since I was fifty years old. I have normalized my BP with The Code of Life.

Whether you have high or low BP, dissolve deposits of calcium, salts, and cholesterol in blood vessels, including vessels in the brain, neck, lover limb (there are some examples below), and in your aorta and aortic arch. Restore your blood vessels' elasticity and flexibility with a request. Check the Efficiency Ratio of the kidneys' mechanism regulating BP and clean it of pathogens when its Efficiency Ratio is less than 100%. Usually, it is all you would need to do. Check the heart for pathogens and the heart's muscles/tissue acidity if your BP is still high. Normalize it when necessary.

When your BP is low, do the Shaking exercise several times a day. It would slightly increase your BP.

Diabetes is a disease that occurs when your blood sugar is too high. Insulin, a hormone made by the pancreas, helps glucose from food get into your cells to be used for energy.

Medical scientists are guessing when postulate that Type 1 Diabetes occurs when "the immune system attacks and destroys the pancreas's insulin-producing beta cells." *The Code* disapproves of this theory. Our immune system would never attack what is good for the body. Scientists believe Type 1 Diabetes is caused by "genes and environmental factors such as viruses that might trigger the disease," an ambiguous statement. Type 2 Diabetes is also called non-insulin-dependent diabetes. Type 2 Diabetes is an often milder form of Type 1 Diabetes. With Type 2 Diabetes, the pancreas usually produces some insulin.

With *The Code of Life Communications and System of Heath,* we learn about several elements that must be checked for genetic damage and the presence of pathogens and their efficiency ratio to determine the reason for diabetes.

1. Pancreas,
2. Hormone (insulin) made by the pancreas
3. Beta-cells

Mike, 44, has type 1 diabetes. His pancreas' efficiency ratio at insulin production is 15%, and he is using some equipment. What is the reason for such low production?

a. The pancreas is invaded by fungus.
b. A hormone (insulin) is invaded by fungus and incurs genetic damage caused by fungus.
c. Beta-cells are invaded by a fungus, which lowers insulin production by 85%.

Our procedure to cure this diabetes case will eliminate fungus and increase insulin's natural production to a 100% efficiency ratio.

1. Read your request aloud one time. With the request, you are using your Biocomputer to focus your energy plus the energy of *The Code* on the target.

Being in the state of Love, Oh, Love! I request thy Infinite Power to charge my Code of Life with the full strength of thy energy to destroy Fungus causing diabetes, restore genes affected by diabetes, restore all organs involved in production of insulin to perfection of health, wipe out from my body all impurities, and normalize the production of insulin.

Thank you! Thank you! Thank you! Thank you! Repeat "Thank you" with emotion for about 30 seconds, thus charging your *Code* with energy, which *The Code* increases many a hundred times.

Depending on your energy level, repeat the procedure four times daily (for a minimum of seven to twenty days) with two hours and 30 min. pauses between procedures. If you do not know your energy level repeat it four times to be safe.

Arthritis. "Although generally rheumatoid arthritis cannot be cured, the disease gradually becomes less aggressive, and symptoms may even improve. However, <u>any damage to joints and ligaments and any deformities are permanent</u>. Rheumatoid arthritis can affect parts of the body other than the joints." *Medical science* Apr 25, 2018. This statement is a ridiculous lie. When people do not know, they are guessing, which is ignorance.

The above statement is ignorant. Anyone with an energy level above 52% can cure arthritis in about two weeks by placing hands on the charged *Code* several times a day for about five minutes each time. Even without being charged, *The Code* cures arthritis with its frequency of 10 to the 56 power.

Viruses and bacteria cause arthritis. Virus disorients and damages genes in the joints, and bacteria cause inflammation. The following procedure is for people with 80% and lower Intel-Star energy levels. When your energy level is 80% and higher, you do not need to recite a poem and charge *The Code*.

1. To maximize the procedure's effect, place your hands on *The Code* and read the Love poem five times

(choose a poem in the Addendum). Keep your hands on top of *The Code* throughout the procedure.

> Ah, Love! Could thou and I with Fate conspire
> To grasp the sorry Scheme of Things entire,
> Would not we shatter it to bits – and then
> Re-mould it nearer to the Heart Desire!

2. Read your request aloud one time. With the request, you use your Biocomputer to focus your energy, plus energy generated by *The Code* on the target.

Being in the state of piece! Oh, Infinite Intelligence, I request thy boundless force to charge my Code of Life with the full strength of thy energy to destroy viruses and bacteria in my hands, restore and rightly orient damaged and disoriented genes, and restore my hands to perfection of health.

Thank you! Thank you! Thank you! Thank you!... Repeat "Thank you" with emotion for 30 seconds.

Depending on the energy level, repeat the entire procedure four times daily (for a minimum of five days), with two hours and 30 min. intervals between procedures. Throughout the day, have *The Code* nearby and place your hands on top of it for a few seconds whenever you feel like it□.

When your energy level is high, you may get rid of Arthritis by simply laying your hands on *The Code* without filing a request.

Insomnia. It is absurd to take medications loaded with side effects that would also inhibit the natural performance of your mechanism of sleep. We have a *System of Health* at our disposal. With it, we can restore all that needs to be set right. The sleep mechanism is located in the thalamus of the brain. It malfunctions when the thalamus is infected with pathogens. Check out if genes need to be restored. You do not need to name pathogens that invaded the thalamus; I did it out of curiosity.

Being in the state of Love, Oh Love, I request thy infinite power to charge my Code of Life with the full strength of thy energy to destroy viruses and bacteria in my mechanism of sleep and thalamus and restore my mechanism of sleep and thalamus to perfection of health.

Thank you! Thank you! Thank you! Thank you!... Repeat "Thank you" with emotion for about 25-30 seconds.

In every health issue, pathogens are instantly destroyed by high frequency energy. Depending on the damage it may take days of charging to achieve a complete restoration; our Biocomputer knows how many charges we need to make. You can find it out with the SP or Simplicity methods.

Here is yet another tool you may employ: watching the mind. I use this simple technique. The mind loves blabber. Do not let the mind drag you into a dialogue. Be patient. Completely relax your closed eyes and watch your mind's antics without reacting to them. You will fall back to sleep in no time. See chapter *Witnessing the Mind* at the end of the book.

Our Immune System and Vision

When some cause reduces the amount of energy feeding an organ, making it less than 100%, parasites may set in, and our immune system may have difficulty eliminating it. The lower the energy to the organ, the more particular parasite(s) would set in. It will damage the eye when the immune system is weak.

Masha had a problem: her left eye's Efficiency Ratio was down to 65%. Using equipment, the doctor detected the problem in the Retina and Cornea of the eye, but he could not determine the cause. Most doctors do not care or cannot detect a cause. They do not know about energy supply and pathogens that cause most problems, disoriented and damaged genes, etc. They believe that damaged and disoriented genes cannot be restored. The doctor suggested to Masha an easier solution: surgery, where doctors also are well paid.

In Masha's case, the causes of the problem were aging, inadequate cells regeneration process, insufficient energy supply, and pathogens. Her left eye received 100% energy, but her Retina got only 65% and her Cornea – was 45%. As a result, fungus, viruses, and bacteria invaded Retina, and Protozoa, and fungi set in Cornea. The underlying cause was aging, which slowed the cells' regeneration process. Retina had 25% weakened cells, and Cornea – had 40%.

To reiterate: Mash's aging weakened the cells' regeneration process, which reduced the energy supply to the eye, weakening Mash's immune system's ability to destroy pathogens in Retina and Cornea. A virus disoriented genes in Retina.

Masha destroyed fungus, viruses, and bacteria and destroyed protozoa to increase the eye's Efficiency Ratio. She eliminated all causes slowing down the cells' regeneration process and causes reducing energy supply to the left eye's

Retina and Cornea. She also reoriented genes in Retina in the right direction. Altogether, it took Masha almost nine months to restore her left eye's vision to 95%.

If Masha's Intel-Star energy level was above 80%, she would not need to identify every cause:

Being in the state of Love, oh, Love, I request your infinite power to charge my Code of Life with the full strength of thy energy to destroy all causes inhibiting my left eye, restore all regeneration processes in my left eye and restore it to perfection of health.

Depending on the energy level, you may not need to charge *The Code.*

Olfactory system

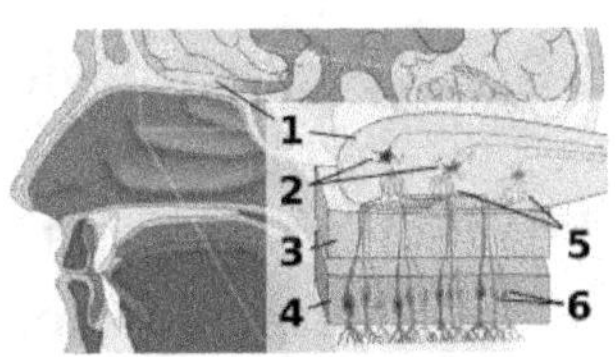

Human olfactory system. 1: Olfactory bulb 2: Mitral cells 3: Bone 4: Nasal epithelium 5: Glomerulus 6: Olfactory receptor neurons. Courtesy of Wikipedia

In the following example, you may diagnose problems in the olfactory system in a couple of ways.

- Holding the SP above *The Code of Life*, look at the picture and ask, "Where is the problem in my olfactory system? Let the SP fly freely along the imaginary horizontal line while asking, "Is it in the olfactory bulb? Is it in Mitral cells? Etc. Relax. You may unnoticeably influence it in the horizontal direction, but so lightly that you would not miss the direction's change, just helping it to keep flying. It may start moving in circles. Let it do whatever it wants because your Biocomputer is evaluating your request. Eventually, the SP will steady its movement in the vertical direction. It means there is a problem. You may recheck it and pinpoint the issue. Let us say it is in # 1 and # 2. Keep going and see if there is another problem.

- You may hold the SP over the picture or the description and let it fly free; ask the above questions. You must get the same results.
- When it is accomplished, find out what the problem is. In 99 out of 100 cases, viruses, protozoa, fungus, worms, bacteria, and damaged or disoriented genes create issues.
- Letting the SP fly freely, ask if viruses, protozoa…, fungus… cause the problem, etc. When the SP changes the direction to the vertical, that is your culprit. Let us say it is viruses, protozoa, and fungus.
- The next step is to recite a poem, ask preliminary questions, and focus your Biocomputer on target with the request to destroy the stuff.

Being in the state of Love, Oh Love, I request thy infinite power to charge my Code of Life with the full strength of thy Energy to destroy protozoa, viruses, and fungus in the Olfactory bulb and Mitral cells of my olfactory system. Wipe it all out from my system and restore the Olfactory bulb to perfection of health.

Thank you! Thank you! Thank you! Thank you! Repeat "Thank you" with emotion for 30 seconds.

Charge *The Code*. Keep your hands on top of *The Code* throughout the procedure

Digestive System. Before charging *The Code,* you must read a poem several times. Choose whatever poem feels close to your heart.

The recital is necessary to raise your energy level. With the SP, you will instantly know how many times you would have to recite a poem. Without the SP, trust yourself to the amount of the recitals; you could never overdo it. Unless your energy level is more than 80%, recite the poem several times. It is a pleasant experience to recite a beautiful poem. Then file your request with Love.

Being in the state of Love, Oh Love, I request thy infinite power to charge my Code of Life with the full strength of thy energy to destroy bacteria in my digestive system and restore it to perfection of health.

Thank you! Thank you! Thank you! Thank you!... Repeat "Thank you" with emotion for about 25-30 seconds, thus charging your *Code* with energy, which *The Code* increases many a hundred times.

Charge *The Code* with great emotion but stay calm detached.

If you do not use the SP, you must say "Love" or "Thank you" with emotion/force for about 25 – 30 seconds to charge *The Code* 100%. With the SP or being a Master of Simplicity, you can learn when *The Code* is charged 100%. If not, give it an additional charge and recheck it.

When initially you were told to keep charging *The Code* with the above request for ten days, you may find the number of days was reduced as you progress. Though it is impossible to overdo it or harm yourself, it is appropriate to monitor your progress. You would often find the initial number of days and repetitions reduced.

Thyroid. In many cases, it is not necessary to remove the cancerous thyroid gland. Instead, fungus, viruses, and cancer cells should be destroyed with *The Code of Life* using high-frequency energy. It may be necessary to diagnose every part of the thyroid.

Being in the state of Love, Oh Love, I request you to charge my Code of Life with the full strength of thy energy to destroy cancer cells, viruses, and fungus in the thyroid, trachea, carotid, and right and left lobe of my thymus and restore my thyroid to perfection of health.

Thank you! Thank you! Thank you! Thank you!... Repeat "Thank you" with emotion for 30 seconds.

Deposits in veins and arteries. At some point, I felt heaviness in the lower part of my body and legs. The abdominal veins and some arteries were clogged with Calcium, Cholesterol, and Salt. You can diagnose yourself with the Atlas of the human body.

Following is the list of vessels in the abdominal part of the body that need to be taken care of: Portal vein, Gastral Duodenal, Abdominal aorta, Porta's vein, Left gastric vein, Spleen vein, Esophagus, Proper hepatic artery, Splenic vein,

Major and Minor Duodenum Papilla, Superior Mesenteric vein. To dissolve the deposits, I had to charge *The Code* four times a day for eleven days. This number of days has been reduced to five days in the process. Later I discovered naming vessels was not always necessary. It was sufficient to name the region. Without Atlas and the SP, I would not be able to identify areas, veins, and arteries that needed to be cleansed. Now I do not need the SP as I use the Simplicity method.

Schizophrenia. Medical science says, "There are more than 200,000 cases of schizophrenia per year in the US. Treatment can help, but <u>this condition cannot be cured</u>. Chronic: can last for years or be lifelong. The exact cause of schizophrenia is unknown, but genetics, environment and altered brain chemistry and structure may play a role."

Is this statement any different from those of 200 years old when "letting blood" was used by the doctors of the time to cure almost everything?

This statement is but the nightmare of the gray mare in a moonlit night. The causes of schizophrenia are made known with *The Code of Life*. parasites but put them in hibernation. The reason drugs are not made stronger is the same as in chemotherapy. A more potent chemical medication may cause irreparable damage to the body and brain, and even kill a patient. This treatment does not cure but slows down the development of schizophrenia and makes patients dependent on medications for the rest of life. When a patient stops taking medication, parasites awaken, and the patient returns to the hospital.

To cure schizophrenia, we are focusing the high-frequency energy of *The Code* on Pathogens and destroying them. We also repair and reorient genes in the right direction with The

Code. When it is done, neuron transmission, including the four stages: resting potential, depolarization, re-polarization, and back to resting potential, is normalized.

Being in the state of Love, Oh Love, I request you to charge The Code of Life to destroy the parasites invading my brain (there may be a need to name parasites,) to restore regeneration process in my brain, wipe contaminants out of my system together with dead cell, and restore my brain to perfection of health, as it was 20 years ago. (If you were healthy at that time.)

Thank you! Thank you! Thank you! Thank you!... Repeat "Thank you" with emotion for 30 seconds'

When parasites were gone and genetic makeup healed, Helen had to stay on medications for six months longer, gradually discarding them one by one, and continue restoring the brain with the above request, filed once a day. Afterward, Hellen felt she was cured. Then, there were 18 months without medications and filing a request, which confirmed full recovery.

Restoring the Heart. John B., 73, felt his legs getting heavy and a heaviness in his head. With years, it was getting worst. We determined he had 28% of his legs' arteries and veins clogged with calcium, cholesterol, and salts. His brain's arteries and veins were clogged with calcium, cholesterol, and salt deposits at 31%. When there is no SP, medical science could give us a good guess on calcium and other deposits in arteries and veins of the legs and brain. Knowing there is a deposit, you eliminate it with the power of Infinite Intelligence.

Include your legs in the request. The deposits may take two to three weeks to dissolve. With the SP or the Simplicity methods, you could daily monitor your progress. Otherwise, go by how you feel.

Besides, John had his coronary arteries and veins, and the arteries that run around the heart like a crown, 33% clogged with calcium, cholesterol, and salts. There is no need to name separately every artery, vein, aorta, and so on. It is necessary to identify the region like the abdominal region or coronary arteries and veins, and arteries, veins, and aortas in the lungs. Make a similar request for each part.

Thank you! Thank you! Thank you! Thank you!... Repeat "Thank you" with emotion for 30 seconds.

When your energy level is above 80%, make one request to dissolve deposits in the blood vessels of the body and brain. There is no need to charge *The Code.*

John had cured himself in about five weeks. How *The Code* dissolves the deposits of calcium, cholesterol, and salt is another puzzle.

Every emotional conflict leads to stress that opens the door for pathogens to enter and attack organs. When under much pressure, make a bi-weekly request to eliminate pathogens in the heart and main organs.

With the SP or Simplicity method, you may quickly determine what pathogens you need to eliminate. You could also determine the number of daily charges and days. The immune system performs many of these tasks. However, when your Intel-Star energy level is above 80%, you do not need to bother with identifying pathogens but destroy causes inhibiting your liver, for example, and restore the liver. You need to determine what power to use and whether it is necessary to use Extensive healing mode 😊

A heart attack. With general health's Efficiency Ratio of 97%, a heart attack may still happen, but only with too much stress or a physical load above the allowed. Consult *The Code* as to how much exercise you can do. The numbers may change daily. Never exceed your limit. Some smarties are advising to work out to sweat. Do not listen to people; consult your *Code.*

Radiculitis. Radiculitis is inflammation of the root of cerebrospinal nerves caused by pathogens. When you have radiculitis, chemicals are unnecessary; they are never needed, just as bloodletting, which was recently so popular in medical science, has disappeared. There is no need to pinpoint the cause. In most cases, it is bacteria.

Once a week, I do a sauna. I do it in Native American fashion by heating rocks placed on the grid with a fire underneath. The buckets filled with rocks are heavy, and I use the Mueller belt when carrying them in and out of the sauna. Sometimes, when I got up in the morning, I felt pain in my lower back. I filed a request. In about three minutes, the pain subsided; it was entirely gone in less than two hours. It may take you longer. It is easier to do it because my energy level is high. Try to explain it to the doctor☺

Being in the state of Love, Oh Love, I request your infinite power to charge my Code of Life to destroy bacteria invading my lower back and restore my lower back to perfection of Health. Thank you! Thank you! Thank you! Thank you!...

Repeat "Thank you" with emotion for about 25-30 seconds, thus charging your *Code* with energy, which *The Code* increases a hundred times.

When your energy level is 80% and more, you do not need to charge *The Code.* You could also use the *Intense Healing mode* when necessary. Always check it with *The Code*:

Being in the state of Love, Oh Love, I request your Infinite power to destroy all causes inhibiting my lower back and restore my lower back to perfection of Health. Charging The

Code is unnecessary, as your energy level is sufficient to do the job.

The higher your energy level, the sooner comes the relief.

When radiculitis persists, it could signify disoriented or damaged genes in the lower back. Damage is caused by the virus, as bacteria cannot hurt genes. Then you also must make another request to repair and restore genes.

Clean your brain of worms, viruses, bacteria, protozoa, fungi, pesticides, nitrates, heavy metals, and other foreign deposits, as well as restoring genes. If you are not a Master of Simplicity and do not use the SP, which helps to identify parts of the brain with deposits of foreign matter, then look at each part of the brain in the atlas, place your hands on top of *The Code of Life,* and clean each part of the brain of all foreign matter. Do not be concerned with overdoing it. It is impossible.

Being in the state of Love, Oh Love, I request your infinite power to charge my Code of Life to destroy Protozoa, Fungi, Worms, Viruses, and Bacteria in my Thalamus. To eliminate Pesticides, Nitrates, Antibiotics, and Other Chemicals and restore my system to perfection of Health. Thank you! Thank you! Thank you! Thank you!

For example, when there is a problem with the thyroid, you must repeat this cleansing process for every thyroid part. When there is a heart problem, repeat this cleansing process for every part of the heart. You can see that being a Master of Simplicity or using the SP would drastically shorten this process. Include "regeneration processes" in the following request:

Being in the state of Love, Oh Love, I request your infinite power to charge my Code of Life to destroy all causes inhibiting my Thalamus and restore my Thalamus to perfection of Health.

Lower Esophagus bleed + Fungus
Read your request aloud one time.

Being in the state of Love, Oh, Love! I request thy Infinite Power to charge my Code of Life with thy energy to destroy Fungus in my Esophagus and restore it to perfection of Health. Thank you! Thank you! Thank you! Thank you!
Depending on your energy level, repeat the entire procedure three times daily for a minimum of six days with at least two hours intervals between procedures.

Cold and flu. Determine whether it is bacteria, virus, fungus, protozoa, or a combination of pathogens. In the case of cold, it is bacteria. A virus that could also disorient and damage genes usually causes flu. Under normal circumstances, the immune system would take care of the problems, but healing will occur much faster with *The Code*. You would need no shots or medications.

Recite a poem of your choice four times,
Read the request with emotion once:

Being in the state of Love, Oh Love, I request thy Infinite power to destroy bacteria in my respiratory system and restore it to perfection of Health. Charge The Code with the emotion, Thank you!" for 25-30 seconds. Words are not as relevant as emotions. It is important to say words with great, forceful feeling.

Repeat the entire procedure four times daily, every two hours 30 min. (the pause may be longer.) Do it for three days (usually two days is enough). Do not take pills.

I was fine the following morning. Because my energy level is high, it makes the healing process faster.

Before bed, soak your feet in hot water for 10 minutes. Wear wet wool socks, soak and lightly rinsed, cover them with plastic bags, and go to bed. You will be fine in the morning. You may take the socks off in about four hours if it causes discomfort.

A virus in the blood causes skin rash

Being in the state of Love, Oh, Love! I request thy Infinite Power to charge my Code of Life with thy energy to destroy viruses in my blood vessels and restore them to perfection of Health.

Thank you! Thank you! Thank you! Thank you!

Pregnancy. Evolution always moves humanity upward toward a higher level of energy and Love. Those with a heavy load of negativity thwart this positive movement. Hitler, Stalin, self-appointed spiritual teachers, governments, violent entertainment, and media are examples of abstraction. The higher people raise their energy levels, the more efficient humanity's inner progress. Nature encourages this trend with birth control: it only "allows" women to get pregnant when their energy level is above 43%.

There are three main reasons why a healthy woman cannot get pregnant. First, a "healthy" woman is not healthy as she has insufficient energy from violating nature's laws. Another reason could be a shock in earlier years that affected genes in the genitals and brain glands (medulla oblongata and cingulate gyrus). Another reason is pathogens, worms, viruses, etc., in the genitalia. All three conditions can be cured with *The Code of Life*.

The invasion of the parasites usually causes toothache. It is bacteria (there is no need to specify it), fungus or protozoa, or all three parasites. Create a request to destroy these three parasites, charge *The Code,* and go to bed. There is no need for medicine. Remember not to use any dental tools . Nothing should be used in the mouth except food.

Headache results from the compressed and hardened head vessels from deposits in the blood vessels of the neck and brain. Deposits are dissolved with the *Boundless force* of *Infinite Intelligence.*

Being in the state of Peace, Oh Infinite Intelligence, I request thy Boundless force to charge my Code of Life with thy energy to dissolve deposits in the blood vessels of my neck and brain, and restore my blood vessels of the neck and brain to perfection of health and their elasticity and flexibility. Thank you! Thank you! Thank you! Thank you!

Another reason is the hardening of the vessels caused by fungus. If it is the case, add the destruction of fungus to your request.

COVID-19 is a new challenge for Medical science, fighting it in the dark.

We know COVID-19 is causing damage to genes in the respiratory system. We are not interested in details, classification, and definitions. It is enough to know that COVID-19 is a virus; like any other virus, it must be destroyed. *The Code* destroys it with its high-frequency energy and restores damaged genes. Medical science does not believe in restoring genes. In our experience, there are multiple examples of restoring genes ☺

People with an energy level of 80% and above do not need to use *The Code* because COVID 19 kicks the bucket on contact with them. However, people with 52 – 80% Intel-Star energy level could still get infected and have side effects.

Why is the Code being so powerful healer ineffective when the energy level is below 52%?

The Code can instantly destroy COVID19. "You have an insufficient Intel-Star energy level," says Nature, "because you have been hurting others and violating the laws of Nature. Now you are given a choice: raise your energy level to 52% and higher, or you may get infected and die.

At a 30% energy level, the probability of death from COVID 19 is 91%; at a 15% energy level, it surges to 99%.

All governments' mandates to curb COVID 19 are ignorance bordering on stupidity. Of course, these mandates are introduced not by the governments but by doctors and pushed by governments relying on doctors' opinions. 95% of American doctors' energy level is below 52%, with 46% having an energy level below 15%. It is disastrous these doctors are advising governments about vaccination and other mandates. The US's remaining 5% of true doctors are helpless against this formidable force of medical stupidity.

The Big Farma is the murderer with 19% of an overall energy level. All vaccines are impotent against COVID 19 and loaded with damaging side effects. However, as of January 2022, Big Farma's revenue from garbage sales reached over 50 billion dollars.

According to *The Code,* COVID19 will stay in the US and the world until many people with deficient energy levels (under 15%) die. It will disappear in the middle of 2024.

The Code instead of soap. Lay your hands on top of *The Code* for about five minutes, and your hands will be free of all harmful matter (when the original *Code of Life* is activated in your body/brain system, your hands will always be clean.) From now on, you can use soap only when your hands are soiled. While your hands will be 100% clean of the harmful element, there will still be one-tenth or one-hundredth of one percent of bacteria. To make your hands sterile, it is necessary to charge *The Code*. It can be done in the morning, for *The Code* would stay fully charged for eighteen hours.

Two sons by the Beatles I found extremely helpful:

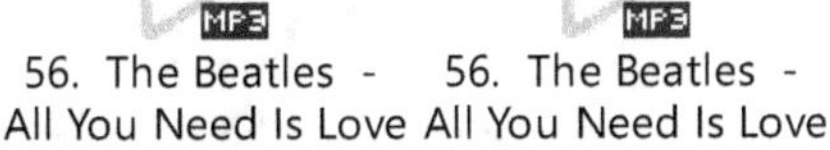

56. The Beatles -   56. The Beatles -
All You Need Is Love All You Need Is Love

Play it on the BG. It would continually remind you: indeed, there will be an answer (or solution to your problem,) when you let the answer come to you. What guys these people were—great wonder!

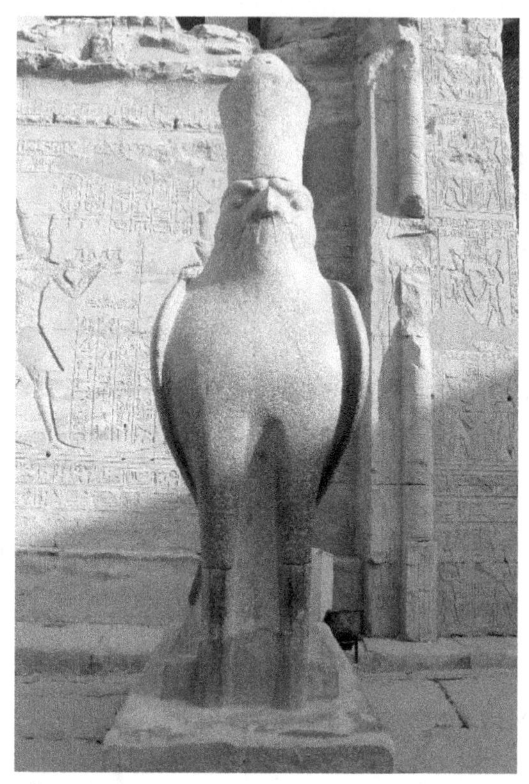

Killing Cancer with Advanced Healing Method

A patient with a low energy level cannot kill cancer. Another person with not less than 100% Intel-Star energy level must destroy it. This person would use the **Intense Healing Mode**. The Patient would only need to lay his hands on top of *The Code* for a few minutes several times a day; the numbers are determined individually.

Always ask if you could use the *Intense Healing Mode* for a particular disease. In the *Intense Healing Mode,* we are filling a request /with fifteen-minute intervals between the fillings for up to forty days in case of stage IV cancer.

Depending on age, energy level, and other factors, you must tailor the number of daily fillings and days individually.

The Code of Life cures any disease because there is no barrier to benevolent high-frequency energy that destroys pathogens, restores organs, systems, and processes, and enables tissue to grow and bones to mend. There is only one condition: your energy level has to be above 52%. When the Intense Healing Mode is used, it can be as low as 40%. The higher the patient's Intel-Star energy level, the more efficient the healing process is.

The Code of Life does not have side effects, as its energy is benevolent and constructive. Only low energy levels, beginning with 51% and lower, are destructive: the lower it is, the more damaging it is.

Every medication created by Big pharma has a deficient energy level and is loaded with side effects.

When we charge *The Code* with great emotion for 30 seconds in the morning, and at night, *The Code's* energy rises to 200% with a frequency of 10 to the 6000 power. We do not know how it happens. However, we know from experience that the Code's healing power and sphere of influence increases greatly with this charge as we can measure the energy and frequency.

With 100% energy and very high frequency, we are immersed in the state of *Oneness* that defies distance and obstacles. No impediment could halt the movement of the short waves of benevolent 200% energy.

You may be interested to know Cleopatra VII, the last Pharaoh of Egypt, had an incredible 150% Intel-Star energy level. Only a very few persons in the past and present have this energy level. According to *The Code,* her body was burned on her orders, and ashes were thrown into the wind over the Sahara Desert. The searchers will never find the place of burial of this beautiful woman.

The Code's healing power would only apply to the person who charged it, except for the high Intel-Star level people who are able to heal others. It is yet another puzzle. When a family uses *The Code*, each member must charge their Code, as explained below. When your Intel-Star energy level is below 175%, you should always have the following Mini Code with you.

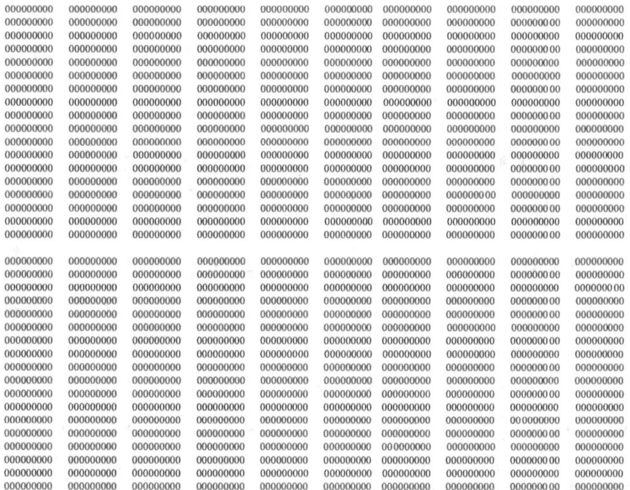

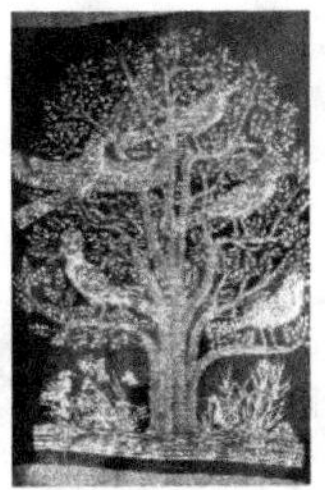

Cut it, fold it, and place it in a small envelope. The Tree of Life has 200% energy and other beneficial qualities. You may also use a picture of Horus instead of the Tree of Life. This Mini Code must also be charged in the morning and evening when you charge the one-page *Code*.

After it is charged in the morning, *The Code* will stay fully charged for 18 hours. Then, charge it again before going to bed. There should be no the mind interference.

While *The Code* is busy taking care of the body and brain, you may file up to three additional requests (up to five requests when your energy level is 100% and more) to eliminate minor issues like colds, allergies, and radiculitis. Additional requests will not diminish *The Code's* effectiveness. When your energy level is below 80%, it is an excellent practice to place your hands on *The Code* for a couple of minutes four-five times a day and file requests.

People with energy levels below 80% should use *The Code of Life* for the rest of their lives (charging it in the morning and at night) because we keep "catching" pathogens and creating ailments unless they raise their energy level above 80%. When we use *The Code* continuously, it will take care of every health issue. When I look at this phenomenon, a floor robot comes to mind that quietly moves about the floor, cleaning debris.

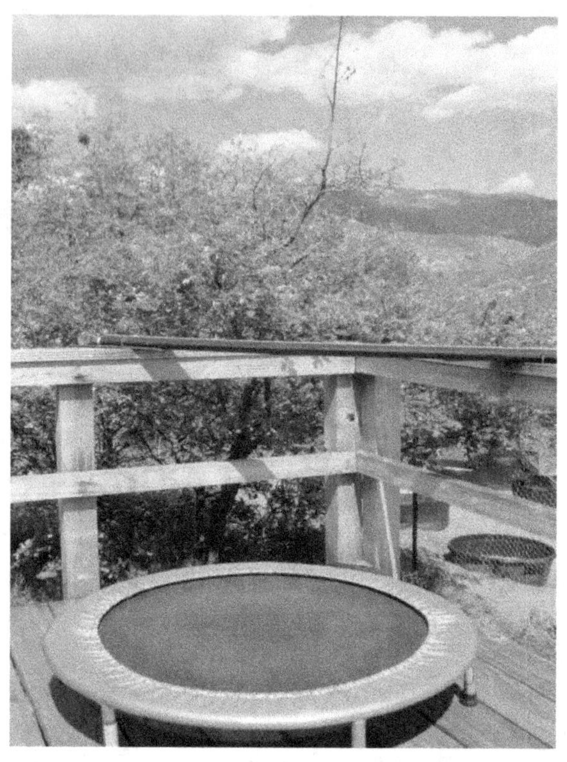

Exercising. With *The Code,* you always could choose what is right for you. A gym with machines and weights is cultural nonsense; it harms the boy eventually. Like splashing yourself with ice-cold water, machines are the way to health problems. On a scale of one to ten, where one is bad for your health, ten is excellent, Shaking is 10, the trampoline is 10, walking 10, yachting, swimming 8, bicycle, tennis, and basketball 3, exercising machines 0. I love hiking, but when I inquired what better exercise, shaking, walking, and trampoline were the answers. For you, it may be different.

Cultural influence often overrides even common sense. There is no mistake with *The Code* as it receives the answer directly from our Biocomputer and Infinite Intelligence that know all we need. First, I do simple exercises on the trampoline. Then, I added a bar, I was directed to do 30 min. training with ten minutes increments and six-minute breaks between them. During 10 minutes, I was doing 45 real hard jumps for three minutes while holding the bar and bending my arms and legs with every jump. Now, at 86, I am advised no longer do it.

Shaking is a simple exercise but extremely effective. I have been doing for years. Choose a branch or inclined trunk of a tree 5-7 inches above your head. Hold on to it with both hands and shake the body by moving your heels up and down for about five minutes. Keep your body completely relaxed, letting it shake well with every movement. At the same time, I am reciting Pushkin's Evgeni Onegin – a good memory exercise. You may hold on to the kitchen cupboard handles or anything like that. If using *Shaking*, you may discard the trampoline. *The Code* "advised," *Shaking* is more beneficial than a trampoline. I suggest to use both. It may be different for you.

Sit-downs. Holding for a small tree trunk or any pole at the waist level (maybe a little lower), do slow deep sit-up. You may use the door handles to do it. Inhale and sit down slowly, holding your back straight. Make sure your back is straight when you are moving up and down. Inhale slowly as you move down. Sit down as deep as you can, and keep your arms straight. Drop your head down as low as possible and exhale. Sit in this position, stretching, as long as you wish. You cannot overdo it. You may also do sit-ups in this position.

Never push yourself to do more setups but ask the SP how many sit-ups you need to do each time. You may be surprised by the answers. A few months after my stomach surgery, I was advised to do three setups, five, six, and twenty. I am always consulting *The Code.*

The best exercise for people with a bad knee would be to stand close to the railing or a tree and slowly sit down (as described above). Sit like this for up to five-six minutes (ask the SP) with your head down, buttocks touching your legs, and hands stretched and relaxed while holding on to the railing. This exercise will help to heal your knees in addition to laying hands on *The Code.*

Pushups. Though it is not recommended for ages over 80 years, I am allowed to do it at 86☺. Always ask the SP how many pushups you need to do at the moment and how many times a day. In my experience, *The Code* was saying "no" to pushups for a while. It happened when I strained my right shoulder while doing too many pushups without consulting *The Code.* Soon, I was allowed to do six pushups for a while, then 15. Now I am doing 15 to 25 pushups and have no discomfort in my shoulders☺

Handrail. It is not recommended for ages over 80 years. Around 7.30 AM, I walk one hour over the deck wearing shorts and a cap despite 8 UV. The Code said it is good at the moment. I have a huge deck with the Red Sea view and the Sahara Desert on each side. After shaking, I do up to 50 (50/50) pushups on a handrail, alternating body weight, and "loading" it alternatively over the left and right hand. Get up on the railing, lower your body on the left hand, turning slightly to the left. Push up the body with your left hand and turn right slightly. Do the same with the right hand.

According to The Code, there is no need for machines and equipment; they are damaging. 10-15 minutes later, I would do pushups on the floor.

Do a very slow and deep sit-downs after finishing with pushups on the handrail.

Listening to your Biocomputer. I have a good night's sleep, but sometimes I wake up shortly after falling asleep. I realized the reason for waking up is always a message. Once I walked up, and after about 15 minutes of wandering, my attention was suddenly directed to my right thigh. Upon checking it in the morning, I discovered 30% Calcium and Cholesterol deposits in the veins.

The next time it was something about a **raw tomato**. In the morning, I was advised a fresh tomato should not be eaten by anyone. Despite prefabricated belief, a fresh tomato does not do any good for the prostate or other organs. It inhibits sleep (about 35%). You may treat it with *The Code* and eat it cooked.

Another time it was **Apple Cider Vinegar**. In the morning, *The Code* advised this product was causing damage to the digestive system. It is not good to use by anyone at any age. All advertising of Apple Cider Vinegar is fake news that medical science has never confirmed. It is the same with hydrogen peroxide.

The above information made me check the value of the other vegetables.

Ginger is the best spice of all. Grounded red pepper is better than black pepper, even red pepper.

Salted preserves like tomatoes, cucumbers, etc., are not recommended for anybody.

Millet and Oatmeal when processed (including steel-cut oats) have only a 5% benefit.

Natural unprocessed oats and millet are healthy.

Unlike nutritionists' opinion, fruits are more effective at bodybuilding than vegetables. You need to check out what fruits are good for you.

Check if garlic is right for you and any other vegetable. You may be surprised by the results. **Wheatgrass juice** is <u>harmful</u>

Except for Carrots that can be eaten cooked or raw, and cucumbers, almost every other vegetable that grows in the ground has toxins and must be either cooked or discarded:

Beets should not be eaten, whether cooked or raw, despite having a 100 energy level. **Onions** <u>must</u> be cooked. **Peanuts** can be eaten only roasted. It is better to use other nuts and avoid peanuts. **Turnip, Radishes,** and **Pumpkin** should not be consumed in any form. They are highly toxic. But pumpkin seeds are good food.

Cabbage is good in any form.

Fenugreek, a white-flowered herbaceous plant of the pea family, is excellent food. It should be consumed raw and as a tea. It is the most beneficial when it is consumed raw:

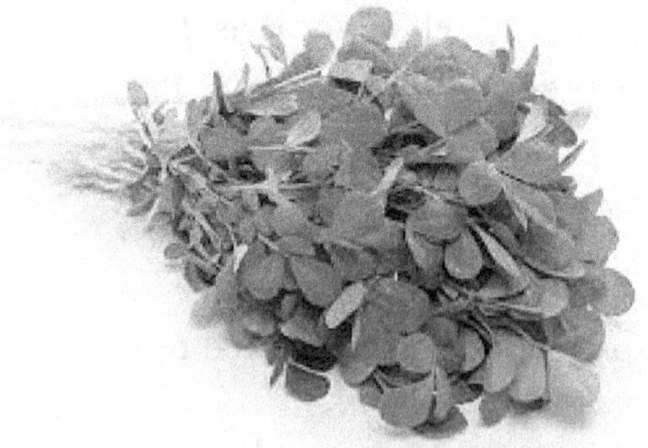

Contaminants can be neutralized or destroyed with *The Code.*

Watercress is another wonderful plant. Use it with Parsley instead of leafy salads.

Parsley is good to eat raw. Parsley is even more potent than Gotu kola and Lingzi

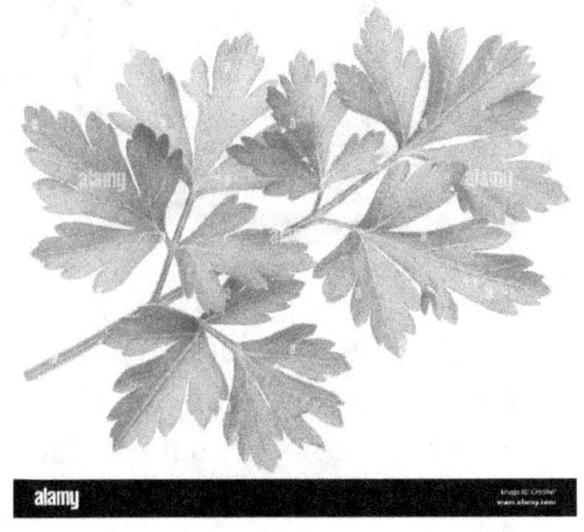

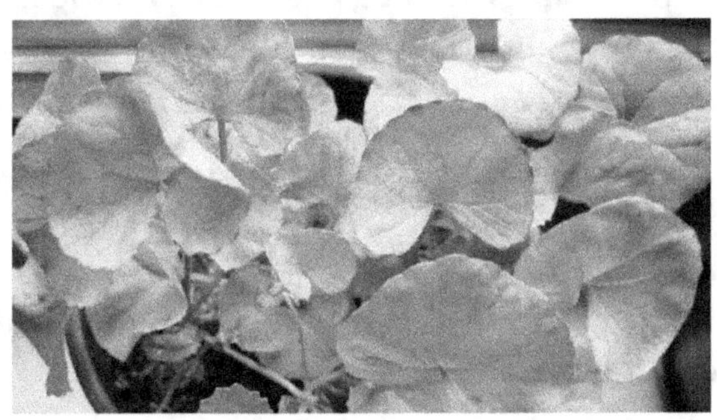

Gotu Kola is excellent food. Gotu kola (Centella Asiatica) has been used to treat many conditions for thousands of years in India, China, and Indonesia. It was used to heal wounds, improve mental clarity, and treat skin conditions such as leprosy and psoriasis. Parsley is even better than Gotu Kola in every respect

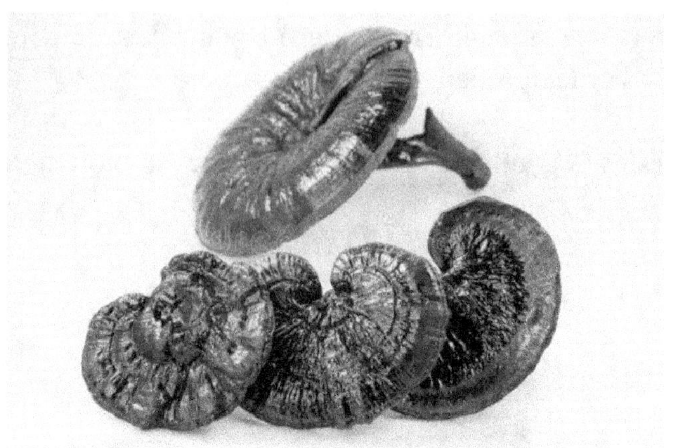

Scribbles scribble, "the name Lingzi represents a combination of spiritual potency and essence of immortality, and is regarded as the "herb of spiritual potency," symbolizing success, well-being, divine power, and longevity." None of these is true. However, Lingzi, a woody mushroom, is highly regarded in traditional medicine, and is widely consumed because it promotes health and longevity, lowers the risk of cancer and heart disease, and boosts the immune system.

Cannabis means Cancer

Like Ozone propaganda, the following information is an example of ignorance and fraud:

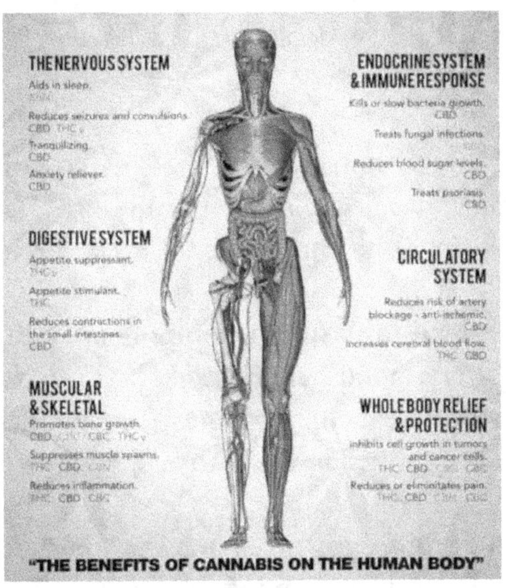

Courtesy of Patients for Medical Cannabis.

The Code confirms cannabis can do nothing of what is said in the picture. Cannabis oil is an effective painkiller. According to *The Code*, cannabis oil would also advance cancer. *The Code* is the most effective painkiller because we identify and eliminate the cause of pain with it.

Black Egyptian tea is not good to drink. Coffee is good, but only pure coffee with no milk or cream. Sugar can be used depending on *The Code*. Dates are the best mate for your coffee, honey, and sugar (for some people). Check it with your *Code*.
Green tea (leaves,) is excellent.

Alcohol in any form (wine, beer, or alcohol) is poison for the liver, regardless of what the wine sellers and doctors say.

Unfortunately, many doctors say whatever they have been paid for.

Avocados should not be consumed. It has toxins inhibiting stomach microflora, vision, and the brain. The toxins are so potent they cannot be eliminated with *The Code*. Research it.

A teaspoon or a tablespoon of honey up to three times a day after a meal is a good health booster. Check it out if you are eligible for this treat. In most the US supermarket honey has synthetic honey added to it. Always check it with *The Code*.

Milk, honey, and eggs are among the best food. If you are allergic to any of it, determine why and eliminate the reason. *The Code of Life* is the best to use here because you will eliminate all causes without identifying them. Only people with 80% Intel-Star energy level and higher may use the "destruction of causes" method. All others would need to identify every single cause and eliminate it. It can all be done in the same request.

Dishwashing soaps are poison. Never use it. It leaves an invisible film of chemicals on your dishes that you digest along with food. Use only hot water in a dishwasher. Even if a tiny layer of fat is left on dishes, it is harmless. You could always check it out with *The Code*. Choose health over looks.

Sun: as much as The Code suggests, which means a lot.

Stress is a killer. Stress may gobble up to 90% plus your energy, leaving you feeling drained. The higher your Intel-Star energy level, the more physical energy you have because you will make more right choices. Remember that the Intel-

Star energy level only demonstrates a person's goodness and vice; it is not physical energy.

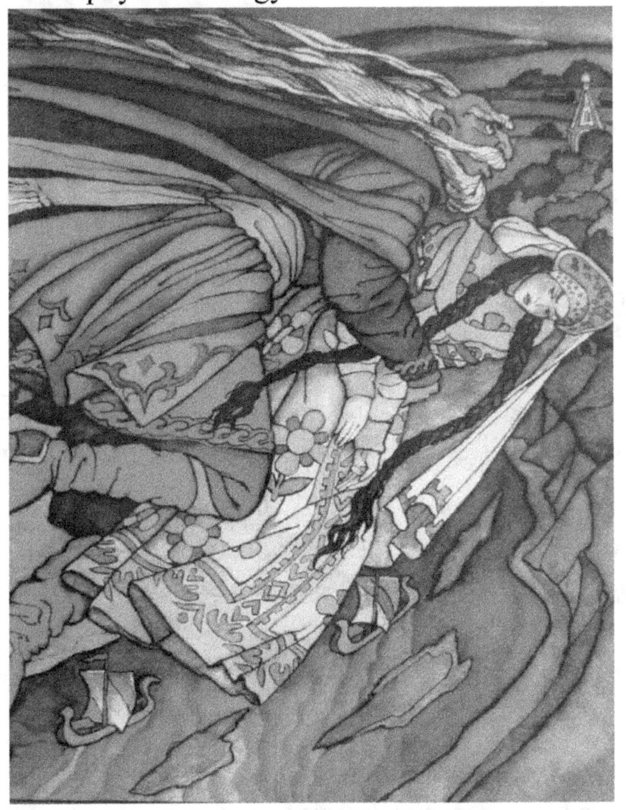

Anna and Nadezhda Balzhak

Poems
By Omar Khayyam

Ah, Love! Could thou and I with Fate conspire
To grasp the sorry Scheme of Things entire,
Would not we shatter it to bits – and then
Re-mold it nearer to the Heart Desire!

Ah, the moon of my delight, who knows no wane.
The Moon of Heaven is rising once again:
How often hereafter rising shall she look
Through the same garden after me – in vain!

Which of the following two poems would you choose?

The spring should never vanish with the rose!
That Youth's sweet-scented manuscript should never close!
The Nightingale that in the branches sang,
Ah, whence and whither flown again, and back returns!
Adaptation by YS

The worldly hope men set their hearts upon
Turns ashes – or it prospers, and anon,
Like snow upon the desert's dusty face
Lighting a little hour or two – is gone.

Oh, come with old Khayyam and leave the wise
To talk; one thing is certain, that time flies;
One thing is certain, and the rest is lies;
The flower that once has blown forever dies.

From the hassle and vanity into the world unknown,
By the enchanted road, over the mountains blue,
Over the lakes and flowers and mysterious valleys,
Suddenly! The world of Love will open to you.
Y.S. Yuri's Hill, Sierra Mountains

Tao te Ching

Knowing people is wisdom,
Knowing the Self is enlightenment.
Mastering people requires force,
Mastering the Self needs strength.

He who knows he has enough is rich.
Perseverance is a sign of willpower.
He, who stays where he is, endures.
To die and not to perish is to be eternally present.
Блажен кто жизни-любви чашу полную допьет до дна как тот бокал вина,

И кто роман её волшебный дочтет до самого конца!

Ирэн допьёт, Ирэн дочтёт, Ирэн здоровой проживет

Ещё счастливых много лет, до ста семнадцати годов заветного конца.

Believe not because some old manuscripts are produced, believe not because it is your national belief, believe not because you have been made to believe from your childhood, but reason the truth out, and after you have analyzed it, then if you find it will do good to one and all, believe it, live up to it and help others live up to it.   *The unknown*

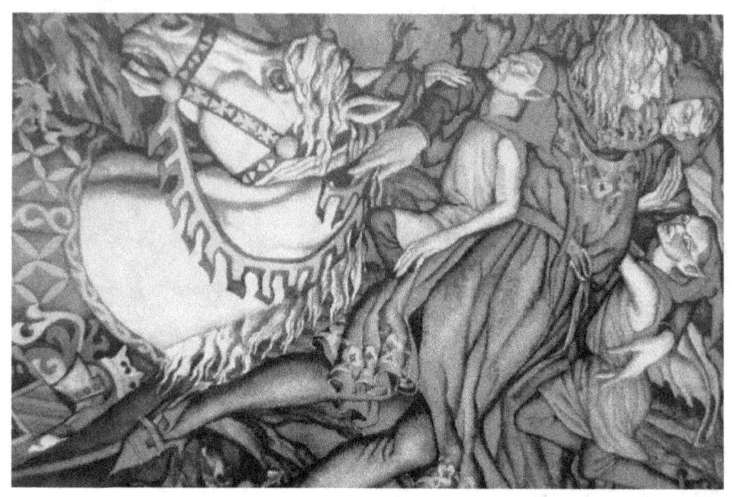

By Anna and Nadia Balzhak

Witnessing the mind

Buddha was one of twelve enlightened humans living in the past 3000 years. Buddha left no teachings; he was teaching with his wordless presence; he was not a healer or philosopher. He was not a founder of anything. Ignorant followers created 32 Buddhist schools with a great number of practices. None of these schools and practices would ever help you to happiness, fulfillment, and freedom, as they were created by the unaware. It reminds you once again: the sooner you become your best and only teacher, the sooner you will understand there have never been valuable teachings and teachers, and the sooner you will find the Truth.

Witnessing the mind and loving yourself is all you need to become your best teacher and doctor. It will bring you to an understanding of the world's spiritual fraud. It is also beneficial in everyday life because it sets us up in the present moment and leads to natural mind control. The key word here is Natural. Witnessing the mind can be done only in the present. When witnessing becomes your natural state, there will be no more effort. A silent intuitive part of the mind would watch the emotional thinking process (ETP) naturally leading you to be in the present, live each present moment completely, and fully enjoy every instant. Thus, by mastering witnessing the mind, you will also realize another secret of life: *letting the future take care of itself.*

Inner progress can be made when you master witnessing the mind and unconditionally love yourself. There is a difference between witnessing and watching the mind. In the beginning, we are watching the mind, a process that can involve some emotions. As you progress, watching turns into a calm (emotionless) witnessing, and you become fit to the following description of Hui Neng (95% energy level):

In your contact with all types of men, ignore the faults of others. Be indifferent to their merit or demerit, good or evil. For such an attitude accords with the imperturbability of the essence of Mind.

Being *indifferent* means having no strenuous thoughts and emotions. There is no such thing as indifference. When it is used, the word *indifference* is used to cover hidden negativity.

How amazingly timely things happen when we let them happen and let *the future take care of itself.* We let it happen when we are loving and peaceful, when our energy level is high and love leads us. Download song Let it Be by the Beatles and play it all day on background. It has high energy and a great message, which you may not be able to capture immediately. Everyone I met can be categorized as a loving or not loving person. I saw loving people have fewer problems. They are content, accepting, and patient because their energy level is high. People, who have been denied Love in their childhood and did not rediscover it in their adult life, have low energy levels; they are irritable, impatient, often getting angry, and have no contentment.

The resistance of *The Code of Life* is the resistance of Love. The limited mind has been our guide for such a long time. It made us a subject to itself. It does not want to give up control, for it trusts nothing but itself. One reason the mind resists choosing Love's guidance is our thinking habit: we love to think and hate it when the mind keeps thinking on its own and we cannot control it. When our energy level is high, Love communicates its message via intuition – another wonder to the limited mind.

When our energy level is high, we naturally, effortlessly, let the future take care of itself. The idea of the future taking care of itself seems strange to the persons caught up in their limited minds. With low energy, the mind becomes obsessed with trying to exert control over the uncontrollable.

A drop of the sea carries within it all the sea. Each present moment has within it all life. It is forever old because it holds our entire past. It is forever young as it looks forward to the future. When the negative subconscious past is gone, our energy level rises, *we live each present moment completely, let the future take care of itself,* and experience life's wholeness.

Society teaches pushing and striving, which is the only thing left to do when the energy level is low. There is a big difference between using force and applying strength. When the energy level is high, society is left behind, and it can no longer influence us. Force is of the ego, while strength is of Love. *Mastering others requires force*, says the Tao (140% energy level). *Mastering the self needs strength.*

Watch the mind without reacting to thoughts and feelings, as if you are *watching* someone else's mind or watching the train passing by. It is simple. Consistently remind yourself of the *watching*. Soon you will notice how gaps of quiet in between your thoughts increase. Watch the mind until *watching* becomes as effortless as breathing. By this time, you will know your mind well.

Raise your energy level, and with practice, the mind will begin to witness itself without any effort. You will effortlessly and instantly let go/transform into Love any negative thought and emotion. It is that simple: decide to watch and continue watching, watching, and watching, that is all.

Learning how to watch the mind may be likened to riding a bicycle. It seems very difficult to ride on two wheels until we begin to practice. Once we learn how to ride, it becomes natural; we never think about it again. It is the same as witnessing the mind. First, it seems a strange and difficult thing to do. As you begin practicing, the ease and benefits of witnessing become manifest.

Always remain in the present. No matter what is happening in your inner and outer world, stay in the present moment. Do not follow your mind's movement to the past or future. Just watch it. There is a big difference between daydreaming and witnessing the mind.

For example, *nostalgia* is negative because it makes you idle in the past. It also adds a sort of "sweet sadness" to the experience and makes you regret or enjoy some things you did. When you are witnessing *nostalgia,* it will show what needs to be transformed into Love. When your energy level is high, witnessing alone will dissolve *nostalgia.*

The mind is naturally empty, and only when it remains empty, without grasping and rejecting, can it respond to natural things without prejudice. It should be like a river gorge with a swan flying overhead. The river has no desire to retain the swan, yet its passing is traced by its shadow without any omission. Another example: a mirror will reflect things perfectly, whether beautiful or ugly. It never refuses to show a thing; nor does it retain it after it is gone. The mind should be as open as this.

Ling-Ching-His (191% energy level)

Your mind will naturally open at a 100% Intel-Star energy level.

Decision and Love
One wrong decision would send whole life astray

From Alexander Pushkin's *Evgeni Onegin.*
Courtesy of Pushkin's Poems http://www.pushkins-poems.com/Yev805.htm

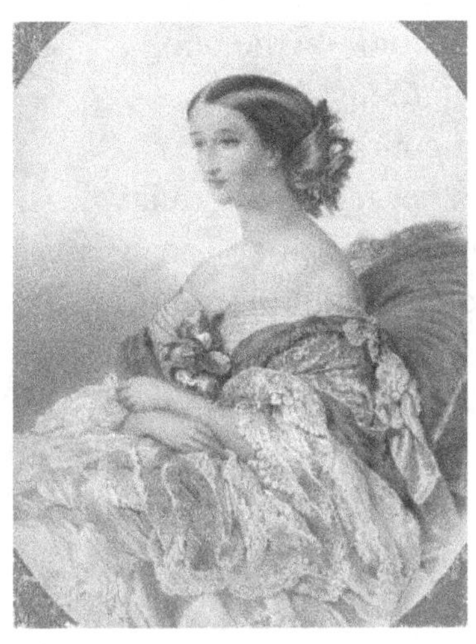

Evgeniy Onegin rejected young Tatyana's love and left abroad. When he returned and realized what a beautiful woman Tatyana had become, he fell in love with Tatyana, but it was too late. Tatyana was married.

But for me, Onegin, this luxuriance,
This tinsel glare of a harsh existence,
My status in glittering society's whirl,
My modern home and evening parties,
What are they? I would renounce them all,
And all these rags of showy pretense,
This noisy sparkle, this rich incense,
For a shelf of books or a ragged garden,
For our old house, poor and humble too.
And all those places, where long ago,
Onegin, I first set my eyes on you,
And for that graveyard, quiet, retired,
Where a cross under the shade of trees and skies,
Marks where my poor old nurse now lies.

Yet happiness seemed so possible,
So near at hand! But now the book
Of fate is shut. Inadmissible
Perhaps was the course I took:
My mother with her tears of entreaty
Prayed me to marry; for poor Tanya
All lots were equal and indifferent...
I married. Onegin, leave me,
You must, I ask you, and I know
Within you, there are nobler feelings,
Your pride and your honorable dealings.
I love you (why should I deceive you?)
But I am given to another now,
And I will eternally keep my vow.

In conclusion, Pushkin writes:

But she, the original from whom
Tatyana's features were first formed.
Ah, how her wretched fate had punished her!

Because Onegin (76% energy level) left, it seemed forever, Tatyana made a wrong decision and married an older man because of her deficient energy level. This decision, says Pushkin, caused Tatyana's life-long suffering. Tatyana's (and her real-life prototype) energy level was 45%. If Tatyana's energy level had been above 75%, she would never make the mistake that caused her lifelong suffering. Unfortunately, with her deficient energy level, Tatyana never found happiness, as her mistakes would follow one another.

If Onegin married Tatyana, it also would be a mistake because Tatyana had a deficient energy level. There could never be a happy union when one or both spouses have a deficient energy level. Despite the initial disappointment,

Onegin made the right decision and moved to Moldavian steppes, which was almost a desert. There, he found happiness. Thus, you could notice our energy level dictates every decision we make.

Peter came to Moscow from Germany, looking for new business opportunities. Instead, he fell in love with 28-year-old Natasha. Unfortunately, Natasha's energy level was 40% (Peter's – was 50%). Natasha did not love Peter. Instead, there was a selfish reason for getting involved with Peter, a well-to-do German, to get out of Russia. Peter returned to Germany, and Natasha gave birth to a girl named Nastya. When Nastya was one month old, Peter invited Natasha and their little daughter to Munich.

When she arrived at the Munich airport, Natasha was up for a shock. A little man came up to her, introduced himself as Peter's friend, and said Peter did not come because he had just married.

That shock was never released or transformed into Love but kept influencing Natasha all her life. Now, well over 60, Natasha convinces herself that the shock is long-forgotten, that she does not care about it any longer, and that she rarely thinks about Peter, now dead. When she does, she is only grateful to Peter for bestowing Nastya upon her, who grew up a beautiful human being.

If that were true, Natasha would not be taking antidepressants for the rest of her life. The subconscious forgets nothing. The shock also damaged some genes in Natasha's brain that could have been repaired with *The Code of Life*, but her energy was too low to employ *The Code*.

Driven predominantly by their desires, people with deficient energy levels refuse *The Code*.

When Peter passed away, Nastya casually mentioned, "There was some disturbance; Peter passed away. Otherwise, everything is fine." The aftermath of the shock was transferred from mother to daughter. It helped to form Nastya's negative attitude toward her father. Seeing what Peter has done, such a negative attitude is considered appropriate in dreamland. Nevertheless, no matter how justified, this negativity does not help throughout life as it would keep causing lifelong psychological harm.

It is an example of conditioning and resistance (the two are always working in tandem) caused by the low energy level. If Natasha's energy level was above 75%, she would never make a mistake causing her lifelong suffering. When a mistake would still be made at 75% energy level because of some extraordinary circumstances, Natasha could correct it. The wrong decision is the cause of suffering.

Decision and energy. People are struggling because they make wrong choices. An average American makes 97% of the bad decisions. An average Russian makes 99% of the wrong choices. A Japanese makes 62% of the wrong decisions. A Hindu (India) person makes 99.6% of the bad choices. An Australian Bushman makes 65% of the wrong decisions. An indigenous person of Siberia makes 55% of the wrong choices.

UNDER OBAMA, the US Federal Government made 99.4% of the wrong choices, and under Trump, it made 64% of the bad decisions. So far, Putin's Government has made 87% of the wrong choices. The Government of Japan (in the past ten years) made 65% of the bad decisions.

What does it mean the percentage of "wrong choices"? When a person makes wrong decisions 91 times out of one hundred times, this person is making 91% of the bad decisions or choices. We do not notice these numbers because we pay attention only to serious errors. The wrong decisions inhibit our inner growth as well as our wellbeing.

As explained in the chapter Key Points, to bring the number of wrong decisions to near zero, we must elevate our energy level to 120%. It will eliminate the influence of negativity stored in our subconscious, adversely influencing our decisions. This cleansing will also raise our IQ, correlated with energy levels. At 120% energy level, we live almost beyond the mind with all its mistakes.

All information on the Internet about Hitler and his IQ is fake news. Hitler was a maniac, psychologically and physically sick person. Hitler was a terrible military strategist; some of his generals were geniuses. How could he achieve such political and military success? Because of his tremendous negative power. On the other hand, someone like James Madison would make outstanding positive achievements with his high-level energy.

The higher the IQ (and energy level), the fewer mistakes a person will make.

Intel-Star, dependence, and religion

A baby is born with a 100% Intel-Star energy level. However, the Christian baptism ritual instantly drops this level to 40%. It is the same with circumcision and Hindu rituals. Such a drastic fall in the energy level results from violating the law of nature as religion initiates a newborn into the world of deception. The other religious rituals, prayers, and worship drop an individual energy level even more, for Life do not tolerate falsehood.

Every religious ritual was designed to control the masses.

Whenever we believe in a lie, a psychological conflict is created. It disorients and finally damages genes in four brain glands, leading to cancer. Religious people have cancer and other deadly diseases seven times more often than non-religious folks.

Whether Jewish, Hindu, or Christian believers, their overall Intel-Star energy level is lowered by the religion to below 20%, which creates the world's major problems because the low Intel-Star energy individuals commit all crimes from fraud to murder to war.

Drugs are another disasters helped to spread by religion. The initial religious corruption that drops the newborn's energy level makes people more vulnerable, and self-distractive because they are now living on the longwave damaging energy. The lower the Intel-Star energy level, the morally weaker the person is, and it is more likely they would succumb to downers.

According to The Code of Life, all religions will disappear in less than two hundred years. They did their job – destroyed many lives and will die out even like more than a hundred other religions kicked the bucket, and no humans would become drug-dependent.

Infamous communist-murderer Lenin was right with his famous saying: "Religion is opium for the people," but this fanatic did not know about religion's ability to turn a human being into a junkie or a murderer. Cultures and governments have also created harmful conditions.

President Obama shakes hands with pornography advocate and "gay" activist icon Frank Kameny at the White House awards ceremony, 2009. V.P. Joe Biden, Congressman Barney Frank, and Senator Joe Lieberman join in the applause. (Photo: Getty Images)

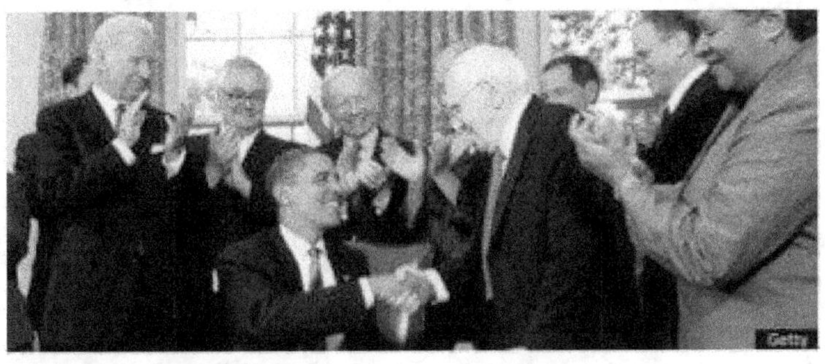

Obama's energy level is 9%; 65 IQ
Kameny's energy level is 11%; 21 IQ
Biden's energy level is 15%; 35 IQ
Frank's energy level is 12%; their IQ is 22
Lieberman's energy level is 13%; their IQ is 22

Pornographic "legend" Kameny was the founder and president of the National Consumers Association for the Advancement and Protection of Pornography. He said, "Let us have more and better enjoyment of more and better and harder-core pornography by those to whom such viewing provides happiness." With his deficient energy level, what this advocate of demise would know about Happiness?

The "legend" kicked the bucket in 2011. No wonder this infamous pornographic "legend" who, according to *The Code of Life,* hurt many a thousand people with his "pioneering" pornographic activity was honorably buried by the Obama administration in the Congressional Cemetery. The energy level of the administration was only 9%. As to the Congressional Cemetery, the average energy level of this junkyard was 11%.

If you noted the Intel-Star energy levels of this "ceremony" participants, you would understand why the US has many more problems today compared to the 1950-s.

Following is another example of the low energy disaster: Mark David Chapman should be given a death sentence for firing four bullets into an innocent person -- and killing John Lennon. He should never be released because he will keep killing. His next victim could be Lennon's wife or one of the Beatles. This psychotic killer had a bad childhood. He was neglected by his parents and hated in school, where they called him David, the coward.

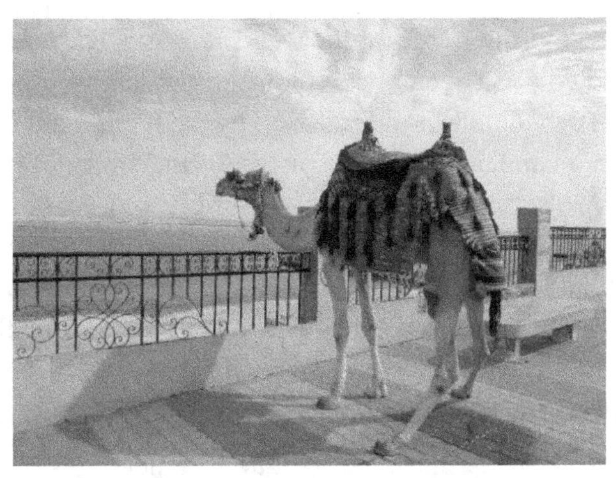

Be your best and only teacher and doctor

It was the cold winter of 1943, the third year of World War II. All frozen, the Volga river was covered with a thick layer of snow, creating an eerie, desolate setting with a fisherman's boat visible far away lying on the side, frozen in the barren kingdom of white.

There stood an old mansion on the high river shore – our home. With its owners killed by communists, the mansion was converted into a kindergarten for children saved from Moscow's relentless fascist bombing.

Along a wide corridor, three little boys were running. They wanted to start a popular game at the time – the war game. They had to steal and hide a huge banner propped onto a long pole to start the game. Crash! Caught between two columns, the pole split, tearing a heavy red sheet of the banner to shreds.

In the morning, children wearing pioneer scarves were assembled for a special ceremony in the large room that used to be a dance hall in older times. In the hall's center, the torn-apart red banner was placed on top of the table and the broken pole. A young woman, also wearing a red scarf, called my name. She said something I could not hear because I was crying as I came in. Then she bent over and took off my red scarf. I turned and ran away as she kept screaming after me to return.

From that time on, I have never joined any gatherings. I avoided crowds like the plague: Pioneers or Komsomol, Communists party, or a church crowd.

We are born to be our best teachers. Life has no meaning unless we find Happiness and share it, helping others find it. When it happens, we fulfill our purpose. We also would help the world's oneness against the negative trends of war, fraudulent governments, violent entertainment, pornography, and other diseases plaguing humanity. It would happen effortlessly when your energy level is 80% and higher.

When you make a permanent decision for Happiness's life to be your purpose, decide to become your best and only teacher. Do not be a victim of self-proclaimed gurus, seminars, and books. Do not get lured by the spiritual industry's promises. Most people spend their lives searching, attending workshops, and studying teachings. It is a useless, unnatural process. Leave the search, and with the *Code of Life,* be your best and only teacher. Reading teachings and attending seminars is a waste of life, for no one ever found Love and Freedom in books and crowds.

To everything, there is a season and a time for every purpose under heaven. You have searched for a long time, and you do not want to spend your life doing it over and over again. No matter how old, <u>every</u> teaching is contaminated with negativity; it is useless and damaging. Enlightened people were a few in the last 2000 years; they did not create teachings. The unenlightened followers made the teachings; it is of no use to you.

Enlightened people tell us the teachings cannot be created because there is nothing to teach about our inner world. Nobody can help you with it. You and only you must make this discovery. The only way to discover it is to become your best and only teacher. You find out it not by learning but by unlearning.

Accurate answers come from within. It will happen sooner when you become your best and only teacher. With *The Code of Life,* you can know the truth about teachers, scriptures, and other information.

You have no choice because you are already your best and only teacher with all the knowledge available. The question is how to access it, and the answer *The Code of Life* is all you need.

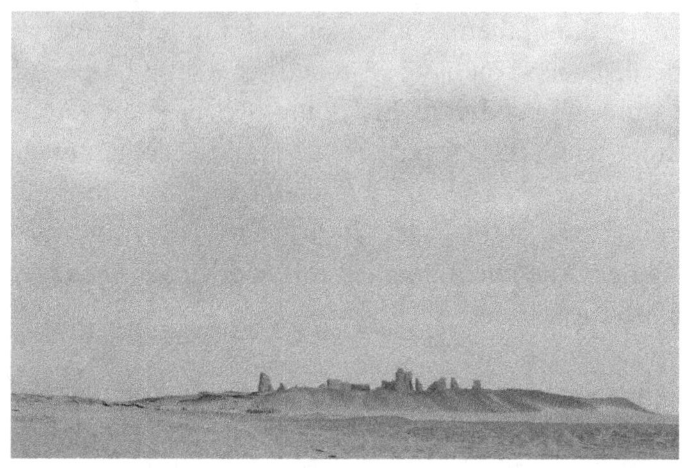

It was discovered in this century. *Blood of the Lion* was a splendid city that flourished over 5000 years ago. Nothing is left of the once-prosperous city: only stones, ruins, and wondrous treasures hidden beneath Sahara's sandy face. Suddenly, the great city was abandoned.

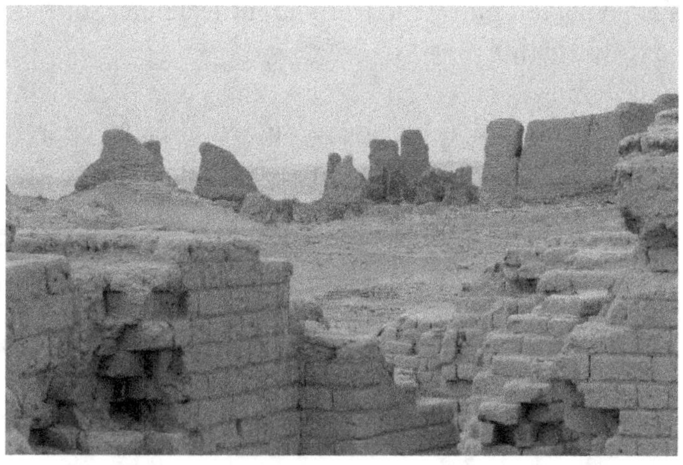

Blood of the Lion was thriving for almost two thousand years to end its life in ruins and be forgotten. There were no names, poems, nothing was saved for posterity – everything is gone forever. Then what was the purpose of this city? Experience of the people: it was preserved – recorded in their Intel-Stars.

The flower that once has blown forever dies

> Oh, come with old Khayyam and leave the wise
> To talk, one thing is certain, that time flies;
> One thing is certain, and the rest is lies;
> The flower that once has blown forever dies.

I was convinced it was an old Sufi fairytale that I love. Suddenly, something stirred within and made me check the story with *The Code of Life*. To my amazement, *The Code* confirmed the existence of the higher dimension! Sultan's story describing his life in the other dimension is fictional, The Prophet's meeting with God 90.000 times is allegoric, but another, higher frequency world exists, said *The Code*. I could not believe it and kept checking this information repeatedly with the same result: The Code insisted The High World exists. "Maybe it is my passionate wish for the story to be true that influenced *The Code*," I thought, but *The Code* asserted there is no interference or influence. See the conclusion of this bizarre exploration at the end of the Story.

Most people live between these two worlds: Heaven and Hell. Hell is reserved for people with 30% and lower energy levels. The world of Heaven is reserved for people with a 100% and higher energy level. These numbers may vary depending on individual data.

"A Sultan of Persia called a conference of learned men, and soon a dispute arose. The subject was the Night Journey of the Prophet Mohammed. It is said that on this occasion, the Prophet was taken from his bed up into the celestial spheres.

During this period, he saw paradise and hell, conferred with God 90,000 times, and had many other experiences – and was returned to his room while his bed was warm. A pot of water overturned by the flight and spilled was still not empty when the Prophet returned.

"Some felt this was possible by a different measurement of time. The Sultan claimed it was impossible.

"The news of this conflict came to the Sufi sheik Shahabuddin, who immediately presented himself at court. The Sultan showed due humility to the teacher, who said:

"I intend to proceed without further delay to my demonstration.

"The sheik ordered a vessel of water to be brought. 'You would see how swiftly a mortal man might travel,' said the sheik and asked the Sultan to put his head in water for a moment.

"The Sultan obeyed the sheik's request. At that instant, the water seized him. Down he went into the water; roaring filled his ears and darkness his eyes. He straggled slowly, as in a dream, pushing against rolling swells; his mouth opened, and he tasted salt.

"As quickly as he was caught, he was freed. He stood chest-deep in the sea, facing a sandy shore fringed with green; behind, the city's white walls rose, set against towering clouds. The air was warm and very still.

"He waded ashore, a stranger in a strange land. But someone awaited him. A young woman stood in the shadows of the palms, a pale, pretty, dark-eyed woman. She regarded him gravely for some moments; then, she smiled.

"You are the man from the sea," she said. "It was foretold today you would come to me to be my husband. I am the daughter of the goldsmith." She put out her hand to him, and at her touch, the memories of his own life faded until they were only pale images, no more than glimpses of a childhood lived long ago.

"The goldsmith's daughter led him into a coastal town, not unlike those that bordered his domain in his world. Dusty date palms lined its dirt streets; behind the palms, high, blank walls rose – silent facades masking the busy lives within.

"'What country is this, lady?' asked the Sultan, who was a sultan no more.

"'Why this is the country,' she replied.

"'Has it no name?'

"'It needs no name.'

"'Who foretold that I would rise from the sea today?'

"'My mother,' she said, with a glance of surprise. 'Our husbands always come from the sea and return to the sea when marriage is ended. Our mothers tell us the day.'

"The Sultan thought of men he had known who had disappeared without warning or explanation. He said nothing; there seemed to be nothing to say.

"The goldsmith's daughter paused by a high wooden gate and rang a bell. At once, the gate swung open into the courtyard of the goldsmith's house. Here, all was shady, lush, and cool. A fountain played in the center of the tiled court, and at the fountain's edge, the goldsmith stood, a tall man robed in fine white linen. He greeted the Sultan with equanimity; indeed, his words had the ring of ritual. 'Welcome, my son from the sea,' he said.

"Thus, was the Persian ruler received into a family in a world he did not know. He accepted his lot – and indeed, his lot was not a hard one. The woman he married was beautiful, and her lure was gentle; the goldsmith was himself a rich man, and the quarters he had for his daughter and son-in-law were airy rooms opening onto the courtyard.

"So, the Sultan married the goldsmith's daughter, according to the country's custom, and he took up his father-in-law's craft: the crucible and the anvil of the goldsmith replaced the spear and sword of Sultan's youth.

"He was happy in that place. After a year, his wife bore him a daughter as dark-eyed as she. By the time the girl was walking, another had been born. His wife had a third child a year later, but this child died. Birth killed the mother.

"After the wails of mourning were stilled, late on an afternoon when his daughters were quiet in the care of their nurses, the young widower stood alone in the courtyard, spent with sorrow and numb with grief. A step sounded on the tiles; he raised his eyes to meet his father-in-law's gaze.

"'The gate stands open, son of the sea,' the goldsmith said.

"The younger man understood that, by the custom, he must seek his death. He nodded slowly. Then he walked out of the gate and into the town's dusty streets. No one appeared. No voice called farewell to him. Through the bordering palms, he walked across the hot sand. Without hesitation, he waded into the welcoming sea, which tugged at his robes, drawing him onward until the waters closed over his head. He raised his face to catch the last of the light. When he did so, he saw not watery shafts but the stone walls of his youth's palace, exactly as he had left it years before; even the patches of sun on the floor were the same.

"Across from him, the dim eyes of the sheik met his own.

"'Have you journeyed long, lord?' the old man asked.

"'For many years.'

"'For seconds only,' said the sheik. 'For the space between one breath and the next. There are places where time marches to a different rhythm. Thus, you can see anything can happen. What is important is the significance of the happening. In your case, there was one kind of significance. In the case of the Prophet, there was another kind.'"

Then what is so significant about *The Code*, I thought. The answer came instantly: "*The Code* is at the core of all life. When it is discovered and used consciously, it puts us at the helm of life, making it a truly happy, healthy, and prosperous experience."

What country the Sultan had entered through the water in the golden bowl, he could not say. He never found it, nor did he ever learn the fate of the children he had fathered. He knew from his adventure that another world besides his own existed, a world whose patterns and rules were different and where he had been allowed no more than the briefest sojourn. He had returned only with memories and a longing that never left him.

Such ventures as the Sultan's were not uncommon once. Tale after tale was told of men and women who crossed the boundaries of their world into the lands most folks had not even dreamed of; tale after tale recorded the incursions of otherworldly beings onto the solid-seeming ground held by humankind.

The passageways between the worlds were always shifting, and the tales always had a nostalgic tone. The old lands were disappearing quickly; the gateways between them in the new, human-ruled Earth were shutting. For all the danger, adventurers sought the lands of enchantment while they could. And for many centuries, those lands were accessible, glimmering at the edge of inner vision, just over the horizon, or hidden but capable of being found. A hundred percent of the energy level is necessary to discover the lands.

When I asked *The Code* to travel to The High World, the reply was negative. The reason is I would not come back because the body would die. When could I go? At the time of death:)

I checked if the other dimension exists and discovered it does vibrate with frequencies ranging from 10 to the 67 power to 10 to the 110 power. In comparison, our world frequency ranges from zero power (death) to 10 to the 67 power (Enlightenment). The 10 to the 67 power frequency exists in both worlds, creating a bridge that makes it possible to journey from our world to The High World at the time of death. However, nobody has ever used this bridge. I did not investigate the true reason for its existence.

Does it sound like a fairytale? Only this fairytale is real. I asked *The Code*, could reincarnation be real? The reply was negative. Is there Infinite Intelligence? Affirmative. I kept checking.

Was the Prophet "taken from his bed"? Negative. It was a mental journey. How real is *The High World*? It is more real than this world. How real was The Prophet's experience? It was as real as any mental journey by a person of high energy level. Did The Prophet connect to *The High World*? Negative. Did The Prophet connect to the unknown state of **Infinite Intelligence**? Affirmative. Is there life after death? Negative. Is there Paradise or Hell? Negative. Is there some unknown existence after death? Affirmative.

My further research confirmed *The High World* is beyond our mentality. Also, there is an Intel-Star, that science cannot discover because of its high frequency. This something leaves the body at the time of death, carrying our life experience to The High World.

The High World does not exist from an average person's perspective but beyond our perspective. No oceans, mountains, clouds, or sky; there is no physical nature. Enlightened beings communicated this information to Brahmins over seven thousand years in the past. Having low energy levels, Brahmins misinterpreted the great message.

From that Hindu mistake, all other religions were born. Indian people have the lowest overall energy level, below 52%, while American people have over 65%, and Russian people have 61%.

Is there proof of *The High World* vibrating with 10 to the 67 power frequencies to 10 to the 110 power? Science cannot prove it because it cannot detect such high frequencies. According to *The Code of Life, The High World* will never be proven. One reason is that it is unnecessary; another – it may be harmful. When someone becomes desperate and tired of living, knowing The High World is true, suicide will be an easy way out.

There is indirect proof. Many historical events have been confirmed by science; some personalities we also confirm with *The Code*. For example, there lived once upon a time Tsar Solomon, says the science. *The Code* confirms it. There are numberless examples of such conformations.

Our energy level must be 85% and more to use *The Code* to confirm historical information. Information about dead people, about anything else in the universe, can be obtained with *The Code* because this information exists in *The **Infinite Intelligence***. That is where we received data about the existence of the High World.

When your energy is below 180%, it is impossible to define the purpose of life. At this and lower energy levels, every individual creates their purpose. Some people make fame and wealth their purpose; others – arts and music; others – engineering, sports, architecture, you name it. Most of us believe children are the purpose of our life. But children grow up, and this purpose is gone. We believe when our purpose is fulfilled, it will bring Happiness. It will bring satisfaction. Happiness is an inner state depending on nothing from the outside.

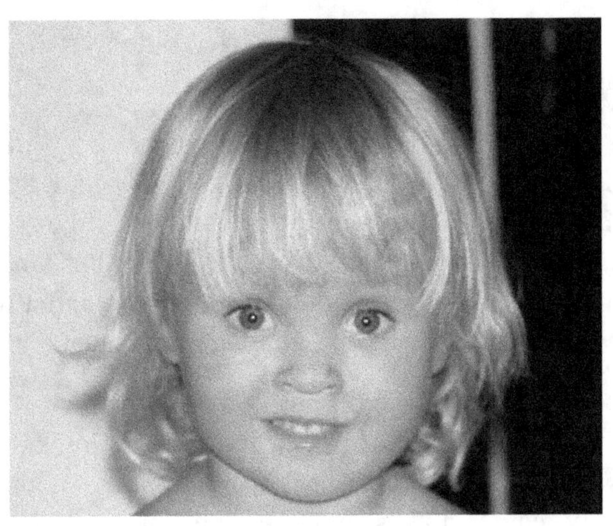

Erenka

I met Andrey and Nadia in Egypt, and we grew into a good friends. They have been married for five years but did not have children. A couple of years later, I suddenly told Andrey that he would have a beautiful baby girl in October. It was in January. Indeed, in October, Nadia gave birth to a girl, and they called her Eren, but to me, for the next one hundred and seventeen years of her beautiful life, she would always be Erenka. Undeniably, Erenka grew into a lovely human being.

Erenka's parents had an average of over 60% Intel-Star energy level. Like every other child, Erenka was born with a 100% Intel-Star energy level, but at the age of four, her energy level rose to 150%; it was 170% when she was nine. She has been brought up with love. Of course, I thought there must be some women with 150% and higher energy levels today. Yet, I know of only one other woman: Cleopatra VII, the last Pharaoh of Egypt. Predictions are not guaranteed, but I was compelled to tell Erenka's story as I felt I knew it even as I knew when she would be born; I also felt Erenka and I have a very strong connection I have not yet been able to explain.

With that 170%, Erenka would make her life of true happiness and success. She would get married at 21 and have two daughters, also lovely human beings. She would be a tremendous artistic business success. Her husband will die when he is a hundred and one years old, and Erenka will follow him when she is a hundred and seventeen.

A beautiful life, I thought, but it is also somewhat sad, for in our dynamic world, who would remember Erenka a hundred years after her passing? But is it important? Another thought instantly came. Life's never-ending unique experience is important only to the person experiencing it. In Bardo, Erenka would have a wonderful time, re-living her remarkable life, and then she would live in the High World of true heaven for another one hundred thousand years. I was trying to learn what would happen to Erenka afterward but was stopped short by *The Code*, declaring it was entirely beyond human comprehension.

We would be OK at 100% energy level. Only 150% and higher **Intel-Star** energy levels will make us truly happy. Today, not many people are truly happy. Then what is the purpose of life? In the beginning, the purpose of life is to be our best teachers and find the Truth. When we find the Truth, we learn there is no other purpose.

At a 100% energy level, the Infinite Intelligence will start guiding us, like it guides the world of nature, and there will no longer be a need for the purpose. Our **Intel-Star** energy will be high, and Happiness will happen on its own. Then, The High World also will make sense to us.

What does it all tell you? Raise your **Intel-Star** energy level; the higher your energy level, the healthier you are, happier, and freer.

Our Universe came out of the Infinite Intelligence that enabled Evolution to develop high-energy human beings capable of making Heaven of their world.

Life does not end with The High World limited by 500% energy and a frequency of 10 to the 110-power. There is another, a Higher world living at 1000% energy and higher, with frequency ranging from 110 power to no upper limit. The Brahmins interpreted these worlds as Astral and Causal. This interpretation has only a glimpse of the Truth and was utterly failed by the Upanishads and Vedas, with their meager energy levels.

According to The Code of Life, nobody comes back to earth from the High and Higher worlds as Evolution never moves backward. We have some vague information about life in the High World. We know nothing about the Highest world. When I tried to make further inquiries, my head became heavy, hinting to halt my search.

The Infinite Intelligence is the Highest World's Boundless Power. It does not interfere with the human world. When at 150% energy level, and only with *The Code's* approval, we may request *Infinite Intelligence's* assistance in aiding benevolent issues.

Being in peace, I request the Infinite Intelligence to destroy all causes inhibiting humanity's well-being.

Conclusion

If you want to find the secrets, think (in terms of) energy, frequency, and vibration.

Nikola Tesla

When you become your best and the only teacher and doctor, your Intel-Star energy will rise, and, indeed, Happiness will be all yours. You would no longer use Love's energy exclusively; you will not need the paper version of *The Code*. You would also use the power of the Infinite Intelligence and *The Code of Horus+* and the more powerful one you would discover when ready.

While exploring the Sahara Desert, I came upon a strange sight. Scattered over the sand, there were black, brownish pieces of what seemed like a stone. Small and large, these pieces had quadrangular forms. Upon further investigation, I learned it was not stone but a million nine hundred sixty-year-old trees' fossils.

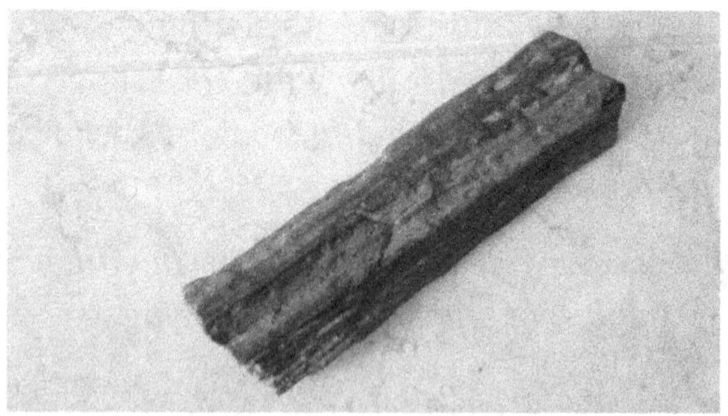

One may discover many strange things in the desert. I picked up several fossils. Two years later, I saw it in my collection and measured its energy level. Incredibly, the fossil yielded 1000% energy with 10 to the 100.000 power frequency. When I charged it, the energy level rose to 5000% with a 10 to the 600.000 power frequency. It was another amazing discovery. How could it be when everything in nature and the Universe has an average of 100% energy? It was another exception to the rule.

While a human being could have a maximum of 200% energy level, advised *The Code*, a physical object could have an Intel-Star energy level as high as 10.000%.

I asked if I could use it instead of *The Code* Horus +. The answer was affirmative. I was also allowed to charge the fossil I named The Star.

For a while, I had The Star with me all the time, and at night – by my side (not under the pillow.)

There was another puzzle. Why was I allowed to charge and use The Star and not The *Code of Horus* + far less powerful? Because *The Code of Horus+* is only a stepping stone to the discovery of *The Star*, said *The Code,* and to the future discovery of the most powerful *Code* with a 10.000% energy level. Eventually, *The Star* was also left behind, but as of this update in January 2022, I did not discover *The Code* with a 10.000% energy level. Nevertheless, I was told it does exist and will surely be discovered one day. Indeed, it was discovered several months later, but in a different form – our 195% Intel-Star energy level and unwavering trust in our inherent ability to be our best and only teachers and doctors.

Please, note that with *The Code of Horus* + and *The Star*, some energy levels demonstrated in the book may be slightly adjusted to a higher level.

When the frequency is 10 to the 67 power, energy is 200%. It is the state of Enlightenment. Except for Buddha, no one has this energy. However, *The Code* confirms 12 enlightened persons living in the past three thousand years. It is possible but would require much time to determine who these people were.

We live in the ocean of the *Infinite Intelligence*. At 100% of the Intel-Star energy level, the receptors in the brain will open. The Infinite Intelligence will be your guide from then on, like in the story of a tiny crab finding its way to the sea. You would become an integral part of nature, living by the *Infinite Intelligence's* power, fulfilling evolutionary design.

You will not need to charge *The Code* as your inherited/given *Code* would awaken (within) and be fully functional.

My Intel-Star energy level jumped to 150% when I decided to drop the "teachers" and their "teachings." Afterward, it was increasing almost automatically as I kept shedding the remains of Yogananda, Yukteswar, Vivekananda, Gandhi, Lester, Garfield, Chopra, the entire spiritual refuse. When my mind was thoroughly cleansed, the brain's receptors opened, and I received information from *Infinite Intelligence*.

Indeed, we die the way we live. The expression is applied not to the physical death but to the after physical death journey in the Bardo state, described in the ancient *Tibetan Book of the Dead, Bardo Thodol*. Discard the book's content about the afterlife, reincarnation, and buddhas. Consider only the travel in the Bardo. I tested this information with *The Code of Life*. It is truthful.

Immediately after physical death, our Intel-Star enters the state of Bardo – the world created by Intel-Star using our life experience. It happens in a different mode of time. The travel through Bardo would take less than twenty minutes for an average person who committed no crimes against fellow human beings and lived by nature's laws. Depending on our life experience, these twenty minutes could be experienced as "eternal" suffering or a blissful journey. Gnostics interpreted this travel as Paradise and Hell. There is some truth in their interpretation as, indeed, the dying person could experience "eternal" suffering of "Hell" or bliss of "Heaven," or something in between these two states while traveling in Bardo.

The state of Bardo is easy to comprehend: whatever experience we had while living would repeat itself in Bardo with one difference. Whether our experience was great or miserable, happy or sad, exhilarating or disastrous, it will be immensely exaggerated. It advises us to discard all the rubbish accumulated during our life. For example, Hitler's fate is to experience this 20-minute-long journey as 250 years of devastating suffering that will never end. Following is an example from my novel *Gates of the Dead*, where Michael, an artist, committed suicide to find his love in the afterworld.

"A magnificent, enormous golden throne stood between the cloud walls. To the right of the throne was a bizarre-looking pile of roundish forms, like a giant, light-brown melons. A light mist slowly evaporated over the throne and walls – the aftermath of what had been in the courtroom a moment before."

I wrote this book in 1995 while studying and practicing useless and damaging Eastern teachings. Unfortunately, it took me almost four decades of searching and practicing to realize that all teachers and teachings must be discarded without a single exception. Only the person himself can teach himself to the realization of the Truth.

There is always a choice that allows living a fulfilling, genuinely human life and experiencing good what we sow.

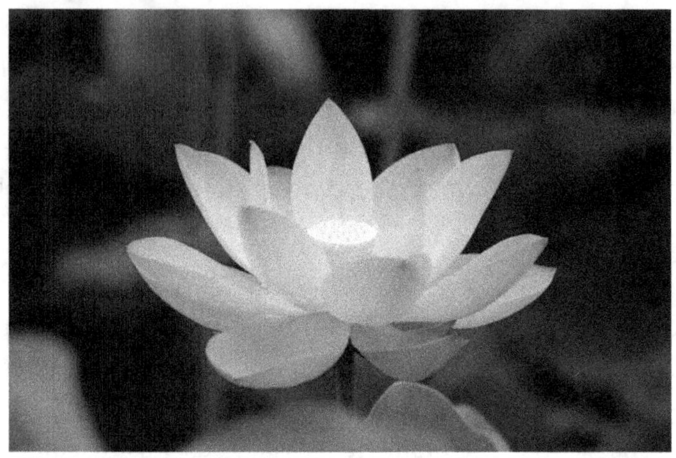

The image is Courtesy of Pinterest

Live each present moment completely
And the future will take care of itself.
Fully enjoy the wonder and beauty of each instant.

Love each present moment with all your heart, with all your mind, with all
your being
and the future will take care of itself in a breathtaking way.

Drop all man-created nonsense and have your life

Triggered by the pandemic and insane behavior of governments worldwide, conspiracy theories are in abundance. With extremely rare exceptions, every government is made of people whose ignorance borders on stupidity. Whether it is the U.S., Russia, India, or Australia, the Intel-Star energy level of the governments is below 15%. There is one exception: the government of China has 61% as of April 29, 2022. It is the same with medical communities of all countries; their overall Intel-Star energy level is 17%, with a corresponding I.Q. 37.

With such a low Intel-Star energy level, the world's governments cannot unite to exercise rigid control, but many erroneously believe they can and already did. Governments act spontaneously and out of fear. They fear for themselves, as they instinctively feel they are the main target of the COVID. There is truth in it because out of eleven million-plus people killed by COVID (April 29, 2022), 97% had their Intel-Star energy levels below 15%. 87% of the killed by COVID were vaccinated. These horrible numbers struck the governments.

The government does not know what to do and turns to doctors for help, which is another stupid mistake, for 95% of the American doctors have their energy level below 52%. These ignorant doctors advise the government, which is always wrong because deficient energy people cannot give good advice. Still, they overwhelm and shut up the 5% of the doctors with the higher energy level who are trying to protest the mandates. And so it goes: stupidity is overwhelming logic and common sense.

Fear, panic, and low Intel-Star energy level throw the governments in disarray. In this state, they make all wrong decisions and do all they can to enforce them, making it look like an organized control. The governments can organize nothing regarding the pandemic. The mentally unstable, hopeless deficient energy government screams to Big Farma for help in its dilapidated state.

Here comes Big Farma, greedy inside-out fraud. Its staff has a disastrous 17% Intel-Star energy level and can do nothing but harm.

It is the same with people who call themselves doctors. In the U.S., for example, only 5% of all doctors, primarily surgeons, have their Intel-Star energy levels above the threshold of 52%. The other 95% are people like Dr. Fauci (9% Intel-Star energy level), whose licenses must be revoked because even with their deficient energy levels of 50%, these "doctors" make ninety-one wrong decisions out of one hundred. Dr. Fauci makes all the wrong decisions. He is the best example of the U.S. "doctors": a notorious liar and palpable fraud. This medical community is capable of nothing and only adds to governments' insanity and the overall atmosphere of disarray.

These disastrous entities are feeding you fake news, poisoning you with medications, telling you what you should eat and drink, how you should entertain yourself, and what God you must believe. Being incurably mentally sick, they tell you how you must live, leading to absurdity, sickness, and demise.

A simple way to eliminate this government and medical nonsense is to be your best and the only teacher and doctor.

To live your own life, make the right choices, drop all teachers and teachings, cultural drivel, religions together with their gods, doctors with their medicine, and become what you were born with: self-confident, self-contained, self-sufficient, and independent of all human-created nonsense.

From Titanic to Julius Caesar

An Intel-Star energy of a human being may vary from 2% (utter ignorance, near-death) to 200% (enlightenment) or a state of ultimate Happiness. A threshold of 52% characterizes the energy as benevolent at 52% and at higher energy levels and destructive when it is below 52%.

According to *The Code of Life*, 91% of all fatal air accidents in the last 50 years in the US resulted from the captains having Intel-Star energy levels below 20%, which also means low IQ and failure to make the right decision at the time of crises. Only 9% of the air accidents were caused by equipment failure.

Titanic. The main reason for the ship to sink was its captain's deficient Intel-Star energy level of 9%. The captain made the wrong decision and took the wrong course.

At the time of WWII, Bismarck was the most powerful warship in the world. The captain's Intel-Star energy level was 10%. Bismarck was sunk in its first battle with the British cruisers.

In WWII, the Soviet army had a 70% energy level. Fascists – 19%. The Soviet government and its military command had a 7% Intel-Star energy level. If it had a 60% energy level, the war would be ended in three-and-one-half years instead of five years; six million lives would be saved.

Pres. Bush Jr. has a 6% energy level and 44 IQ. If this utterly stupid person had a 60% energy level, he would not invade and destroy Iraq.

Obama has a 9% energy level with a low IQ. If this demagogue and a palpable fraud had a 60% energy level, he would not destroy prosperous Libya and drop 135,000 bombs on the world.

Osama Bin Laden had an 81% energy level. A gifted person, he was not a terrorist but was fighting against the American invasion. American "hero" who killed Osama had a 7% energy level.

President of Libya Khaddaffi had a 70% energy level, which is much higher than the US presidents after Roosevelt and before Trump. These so-called presidents had an overall energy level of catastrophic 11%. They were destroying America. In thirty years of his rule, Khaddaffi built Libya from a backward country to a prosperous nation with higher living standard than the US. Obama pushed Libya thirty years back to where it was before Khaddaffi. Obama (9% energy level), destroyed Libya and caused Khaddaffi's murder.

For desert, please have the truth about Julius Caesar. There is 95% of fake news on the web about Julius, like every other famous personality of the past and present. A great character and the world's best-ever military leader, writer, and philosopher, Julius had an 86% energy level. Wikipedia and National Geographic claim Julius was a dictator. Both publications are ridden with errors in everything they publish. With such a high energy level, Julius could never be a dictator. All dictators had an extremely low Intel-Star energy level, and none of them lived by the laws of Nature.

Julius was married to Cleopatra VII, the last Pharaoh of Egypt. They had a son. Cleopatra had an incredible 150% Intel-Star energy level.

Julius was killed not because he "accumulated too much power," as the mediocre historians write, but because he introduced a law to curb homosexuality in Rome. 70% of the Roman senators of the time were homosexual. Brutus, a homosexual, had a 9% energy level.

People with low energy levels have been murdering great human beings with high energy levels throughout history. You can know the truth about people and events only with *The Code of Life Communications and System of Health.*

The Intense Healing Mode

When your Intel-Star (soul) energy level is 80% and more, do not diagnose an ailment, identify the causes, but *destroy all the illness's cause*s.

Suddenly, my arms and hands started etching. After falling asleep at night, I would wake up two hours later, scratching my arms and hands. It would continue for a couple of hours, then disappear. It could start with the upper arms, then go down to the hands, or vice-versa. I was curious about what was causing it. Was it an allergic reaction to mango or some other fruit, or was it some pathogen, but I failed.

I decided to use the Intense Healing mode *to destroy all causes inhibiting my skin and restore it*. It worked like a clock, and there was no more itching the following night. I still do not know what was causing the itching, but it was no longer important. It was not important at all. However, when your energy level is below 80%, you must identify every reason for an ailment.

There are several points to remember:
1. Your energy level must be 80% higher to use the Intense Healing Mode and destroy *all inhibiting causes,* instead of identifying them.
2. You must choose the right energy: the energy of Love or the energy of the Infinite Intelligence. You do it with *The Star Pendulum* or with the *Method of Simplicity.* This choice makes all the difference. It is still the puzzle why, for example, to eliminate itching, I had to use the energy of Love and not the energy of the Infinite Intelligence. It defies logic because the energy of the Infinite Intelligence is more powerful than the energy of Love. I have no answer to this puzzle. Try to guess it and, please, let me know ☺
3. In the Intense Healing Mode, choose the right pause. It could be either 15 minutes or 30 minutes between procedures. It is another puzzle because the pause between procedures must be not less than 2 hours and 30 min in the Regular Healing Mode for *The Code* to do the job. However, *The Code* works beautifully in the Intense Healing Mode, with the pause as short as only 15 minutes.

There, it seems some hidden laws at work because to restore the heart, for example, or reproductive organs, we must use the energy of Love. Is it because reproductive organs and the Heart also are symbols of Love? However, to restore the

Thyroid, Urinary System, and Vision, we have to use the energy of the Infinite Intelligence. Whatever the answer to this puzzle, we must employ the right energy source for each task.

Every secret is told

Every thought, emotion, action, everything that contributes to what we are is converted/transformed into an energoinformational record and is sent to our Intel-Star's outer field. The total of all records determines our Intel-Star energy level. Thus, the composite of all energoinformational records represents our Intel-Star's energy level. This energy level can be verified or "read."

Oneness facilitates this reading ability. In the state of Oneness, everything is here and now; everything and everyone is connected with all other people and objects, and the distance does not exist. The higher our energy level, the more immersed we are in this wonderful state of Oneness, the more accurate our "reading" of other people and diagnoses.

Intel-Star does not influence our life. We do it. Intel-Star only collects our activity records and has them available for anyone to "read." Thus, the old saying "my mind is my fortress," meaning nobody can read someone else's mind, become outdated and "the fortress" – penetrated because anyone with an energy level of 120% could "read" another person's mind. Not the emotional thought process but personal qualities, and have an accurate picture of the person. Every person becomes an "open book," revealing their true nature. As Emmerson said, "Every secret is told." Nothing can be covered or hidden from us when our energy level is 170% and above. Many secrets are told with a 120% energy level; with 170%, all secrets are told.

Longevity

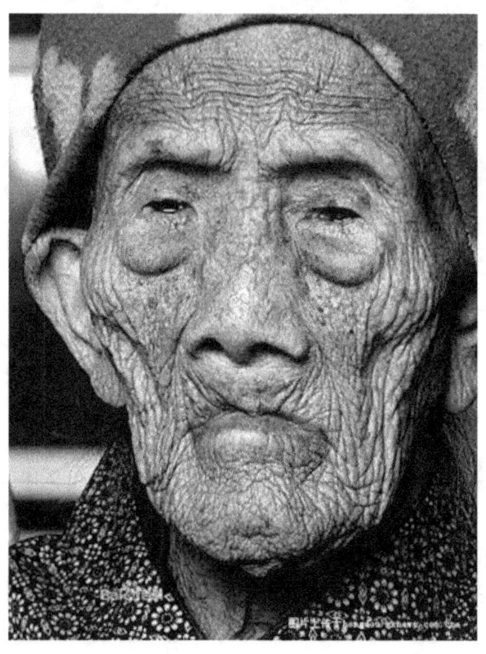

Numerous sources, including Times and National Geographic, tell us Li Qingyun (above) lived 260 years. According to *The Code*, he died when he was 156 years old. Many said Li Qingyun was never ill and died of natural causes. However, Li Qingyun was sick many times and died of pneumonia. Some claim he practiced breathing and physical exercises that a 500 years old recluse taught him in the mountains. There was no such recluse.

Fortunately, Li Qingyun practiced no exercises but loved walking. In the last year of his life, he walked about two miles two-three times a week.

He suggested *keeping a quiet heart, sitting like a tortoise, walking sprightly like a pigeon, and sleeping like a dog.*

He was married three times and had eleven children. He did not eat meat and fish but had milk, eggs and cheese, and a chicken soup once or twice a week. He ate Lingzi, Wild Ginseng, Gotu Kola, among other herbs. Scribbles scribble, "the name Lingzi represents a combination of spiritual potency and essence of immortality, and is regarded as the "herb of spiritual potency," symbolizing success, well-being, divine power, and longevity." None of these is true. It is true, however, that Lingzi, a woody mushroom, is highly regarded in traditional medicine and is widely consumed because it promotes health and longevity, lowers the risk of cancer and heart disease, and boosts the immune system.

Li Qingyun had a 112% Intel-Star energy level with an IQ of 154. He was not a religious person and had no disciples. What helped him to live so long? One of the reasons was his natural way of living. However, many people lived this way in China at the time, but none that long. The major reason was his discovery of how to maintain his health without doctors and medicines of the time.

Step by step, *The Code of Life* brings us to the point when we become our teachers and doctors. So did Li Qingyun. At the beginning of this journey, we are using tools. Then, we realize our inherent ability to manage our health and life exclusively ourselves and discard the tools.

It also happened to Li Qingyun and every other person who lived past 100 years. Every one of them discovered this inherent ability that made them independent of the influence of society, religion, teachers, teachings, and doctors. Each of them has been led by the Infinite Intelligence, thus making fewer or no mistakes. Regardless of the surrounding circumstances, every one of them has been living *their* life.

The following list demonstrates how longevity correlates with Intel-Star and IQ.

	Age	Intel-Star Energy	IQ
Kirk Douglas	101	93	136
Betty White,	96	98	141
Carol Channing,	97	87	122
Cicely Tyson,	94	94	126
Sean Connery,	88	94	144
Tony Bennet,	92	92	127
Eva Marie,	94	97	137
Julie Gibson,	105	98	144
Norman Lloyd,	104	97	143
Carl Reiner,	96	96	142
Rhonda Fleming,	95	96	
Barbara Eden,	96	94	
Ann Blithe,	90	92	
Doris Day,	96	95	
Sidney Poitier,	91	93	135
Bob Barker,	94	91	
Olivia de Havilland,	102	99	
Li Qingyun	156	112	154

Li is the longest living human. He was living in China.

Longevity courtesy of:
https://www.novelodge.com/worldwide/old-celebs-2/31

Believing in a lie

Pandemics appeared on Earth together with humanity 12 million years ago. The purpose of pandemics is to safeguard humanity from destruction. Pandemics infect people with below 80% Intel-Star energy levels. The lower is energy level, the more severe is damage to the body and brain in the future, despite the successful recovery.

Pandemics kill people who have Intel-Star energy levels below 15%. The reason is that these people violate the laws of nature by harming others and engaging in corrupt ways of life and relationships. Making yourself believe in a lie is the same violation of the laws of nature as hurting others and using drugs.

To thwart a lie, evolution disorients genes in the following glands of the liar's brain: Hypothalamus sulcus, Septum Pellucidum, Precuneus, Central sulcus, Stria Medullary of the Thalamus Parietooccipital, Straight sinus in tentorium cerebelli, and Caudate nucleus, which leads to psychological disorders. There are no lies in nature; a lie is created and accepted as truth only by the mind.

When believing in a lie persists, disoriented genes in affected glands of the brain get damaged. Damage to genes anywhere in the brain leads to cancer or similar disease.

An average Intel-Star energy level of all believers in a lie is 20%. Pandemics primarily target these people and kill people with Intel-Star energy levels below 15%.

Talent Happiness and Success

You must have a 175% Intel-Star energy level to be your best and the only teacher and learn if you have *Talent*, such as creating wealth, being a successful filmmaker or designer, or any other *Talent*. *The Code of Life* will take you beyond the limitations of the mind and into the real world governed by True Love.

There is an infinite number of mysteries in life. Our solar system and the universe are great mysteries. Intuition is a mystery. There's also something called *Talent*, which is an unsolvable mystery. Over 130 billionaires, *The Giving People* pledged up to 99% of their wealth to charity. They are *True Dreamers of the American dream*. Many of these people are using the word "luck" as one of the reasons for success. What is luck? By luck, some mean being born in America, the land of opportunities; others believe luck means lucky genes or being born to loving parents. Though all this helps to succeed, there is no such thing as "luck," which word is used when the reason for success is unknown. The success that people believe is luck, in reality, is caused by *Talent*.

Love, imagination, and *Talent* together play a major role in creating Success (with a capital S). Because *Talent* and Love are indefinable, Success has no rules that one can use to become successful. Yet, Love will reveal your *Talent* to you and guarantee Success in any field harmonious with your *Talent*. Being led by Love, you will catch two birds: Happiness and Success.

Only as a distant approximation may we allude to *Talent* as a set of special qualities. Each quality must be uniquely individual and harmonious with all other qualities to create a genius in any field of life. The more fine-tuned and harmonious the alliance of these qualities, the greater success is. When one or more of these unidentifiable qualities are lacking, there can be no Beethoven or Somerset Maugham; still, a rapper may happen or a writer of the bestselling murder mystery. Yet, any individual can discover their *Talent* and succeed in a field harmonious with their *Talent.*

Every Talent is purely individual. Every original (as opposed to inherited) great wealth has been created with a unique individual *Talent*, even like *Gone with the Wind* and *The Razor's Edge* were written by the people of great *Talent*. *Talent* cannot be acquired like skill, for *Talent* is inborn and indefinable.

When one attempts to be successful without having *Talent*, he's bound for a life of frustration. Millions are wasting their time misled by teachers, "success books," and media. When it comes to wealth, the American Dream is a hoax that teaches success without considering *Talent*. A huge "success industry" has been built upon this ruse. Even though there is no intention here to mislead, it is an erroneous conviction, a cultural belief that the art of wealth building can be taught and learned. To understand it, we must be our best and the only teachers

The above is pertinent to any field of life. Practically anyone may acquire any skill, but to become successful (as opposed to being just mediocre), one must select a vocation harmonious to their *Talent*. For example, President Bush Jr. had no *Talent* in leadership and as a commander in chief, yet he was promoted to the White House. The result was disastrous. It happens to many people who have chosen a vocation not harmonious with their *Talent*.

It's the same with wealth. To be at the right time in the right place, sense and exercise the right opportunities, and create opportunities are qualities of the *Talent*. Is it possible to develop these qualities? When a complete set of unique attributes is in place, Warren Buffett happens. When some of these qualities are missing or not harmonious, there comes Sean Hyman, who claims to discover a wealth Code in the Bible.

The truth is Sean is making money because he has the *Talent* to make money. In Sean's example, it's a small *Talent* that does it. Between Warren Buffett and Sean Hyman, many people have different degrees of *Talent*, enabling them to create different size fortunes. Yet, whether it is small like Sean's, grand like Warren's, or supreme like Andrew Carnegie's, there must always be *Talent* to create wealth. No code, book, or financial adviser will help create wealth if one has no *Talent*. I'm sure that from Napoleon Hill to Sean Hyman, success reports and books writers and teachers of all kinds mean good to their readers and clients. Unfortunately, to the multitudes of wealth seekers, it helps nothing.

Courtesy of Thrive: https://thriveglobal.com/stories/a-letter-from-albert-einstein-to-his-daughter/

Psychological Balance

Psychological balance (PsB) is the key to a happy, healthy, and fulfilled life. PsB means inner harmony and balance of emotions and thoughts. I.e., PsB means naked, free of stress, the mind also free of concepts created by others (religion, various groups, and teachers). It is the independent mind of someone who became their best and only teacher.

The mind is in control of the body; it controls our life. The mind is controlled by the subconscious, which, in turn, is controlled by Intel-Star (soul) energy level.

An **Intel-Star** is a unique module that the writers of the Bible call soul. It is attached to us <u>at the time of birth</u>. It departs at the time of death, loaded with our life experiences.

Intel-Star's outer Energoinformational field has an upper-frequency limit of 10 to the 67 power at 200% energy. It is the frequency and energy of the Enlightenment. Its lower limit is "0," or a point of death. An Intel-Star's energy level could drop as low as 4% (Adolf Hitler) with a corresponding 10 to the 6 power frequency, influencing human behavior accordingly.

With some exceptions, the frequencies of the world and the Universe are 10 to the 56% Power (energy 100%), which is the frequency and energy level of what we call true Love. It is also the standard against which Intel-Star's percentage or energy level is calculated.

The nature of the Intel-Star energy and frequency is the same as in electricity. It has a greater frequency and a much higher upper limit than electricity. A person's Intel-Star energy level is the only accurate indicator of the person's goodness and vice. The mechanics are quite simple here. In the outer field of the Intel-Star, an energy level indicates our energoinformational state. It is not used for healing or any other purpose. A thermometer is a good example, as its mercury shows the number of degrees while the total amount of mercury remains the same at any degree. It is the same with the energy of the outer field of Intel-Star.

The core of Intel-Star has a 500% energy level that makes it indestructible. It provides emotional thinking/healing energy. The "physical" energy we get from food. The food provides the body with lower (compared Intel-Star's) energy levels and frequency. The body converts food with an energy level below 95% to fat. Examples are potato 23%; leafy salads 51%; all processed food with not a single exception has an overall energy level of 23%, like all-natural pizza that has a 40% energy level; sugar 75%; all processed, including "natural," drinks have an overall energy level of 31%; Coca-Cola 61%; it all contributes to fat.

The newborn gets Intel-Star of true Love and, like everything in nature, gets 100% energy. However, baptismal or any other religious ritual drops the energy level to 40%-30%. This happens because there is not a lie in nature, but an introduction to any religion is an introduction to a lie because religion is not truthful. Nature has no lies; only the human mind creates lies. But unlike the human mind, which often compromises, Nature does not compromise. It drops the newborn's energy level when introduced to a lie. It is a warning to people; do not lie! Do not believe in lies! As believing in a lie is the same as lying. Nature goes even further: When the energy thus drops, the newborn loses the opportunity to create a happy life in the future and becomes vulnerable to downers, alcohol, smoking, and other negativity.

As explained in this book, we must aspire to raise our Intel-Star energy level to a higher level. Psychological balance is reached when the Intel-Star energy level is 170%. When Intel-Star's energy level is lower, there are psychological discrepancies such as stress, relationship conflict, rejection, judgment, worry, doubts, and so on. It must be eliminated. It will disappear when the energy level is raised to 170%.

When we attain Psychological balance, our SP reading becomes almost100% accurate.

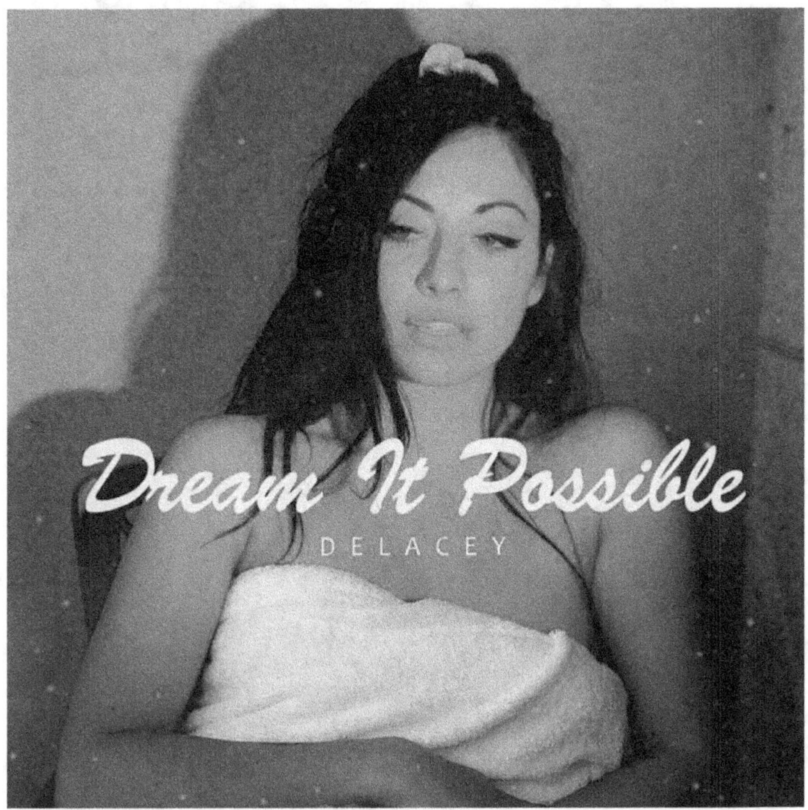

Jan Zhan has a 197% Intel-Star energy level. Amazing and understandable. Dream it Possible is a beautiful song with the same 197% energy level.

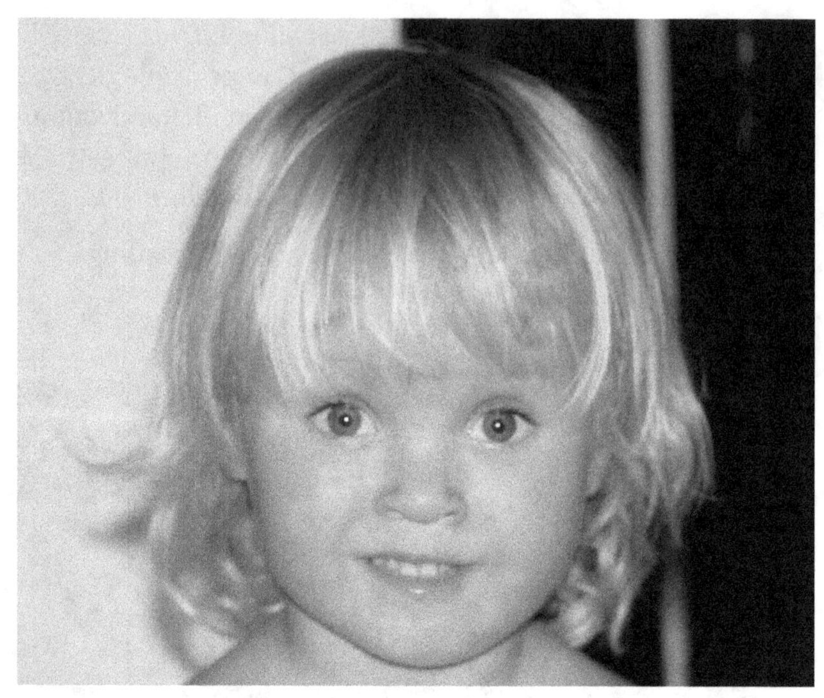

199 energy level.

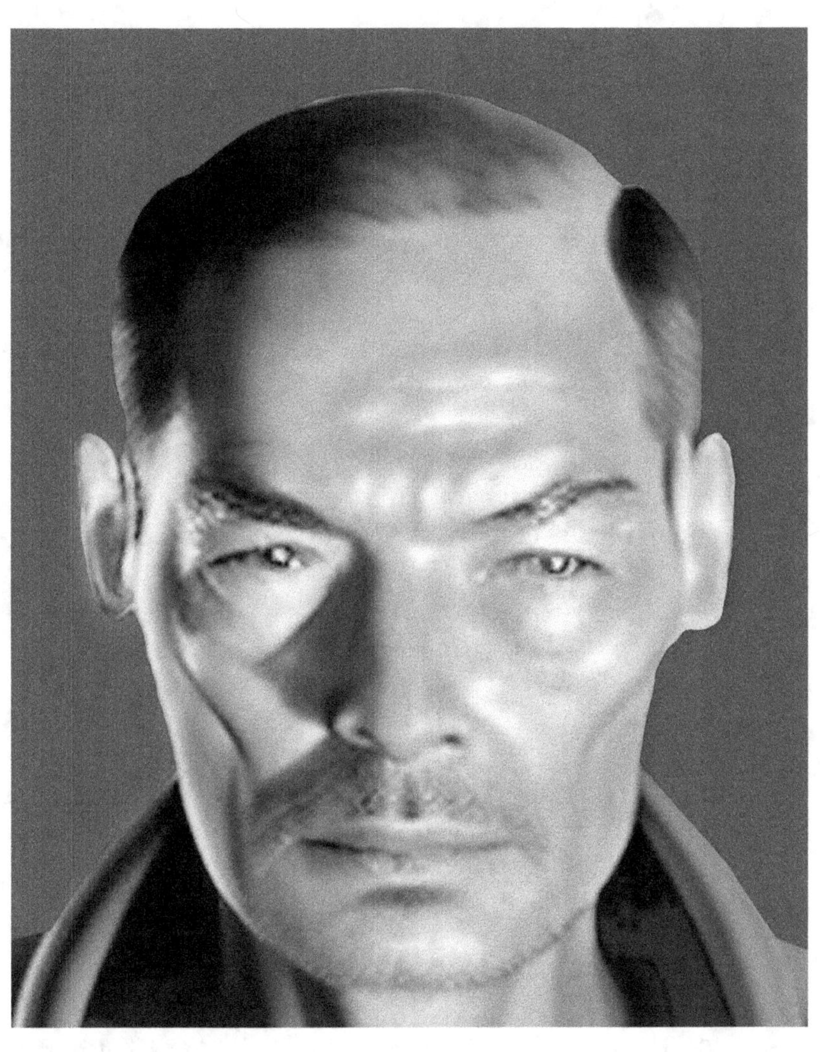

200 energy level

THE UNIVERSAL FORCE OF LOVE

Thrive invites voices from many spheres to share their perspectives on our community platform. Community stories are not commissioned by our editorial team, and opinions expressed by Community contributors do not reflect the opinions of Thrive or its employees. More information on our Community guidelines is available here.

A letter from Albert Einstein to his daughter, Lieserl on The Universal Force of Love

"When I proposed the theory of relativity, very few understood me, and what I will reveal now to transmit to mankind will also collide with the misunderstanding and prejudice in the world.

I ask you to guard the letters as long as necessary, years, decades, until society is advanced enough to accept what I will explain below.

There is an extremely powerful force that, so far, science has not found a formal explanation to. It is a force that includes and governs all others, and is even behind any phenomenon operating in the universe and has not yet been identified by us. This universal force is LOVE.

When scientists looked for a unified theory of the universe they forgot the most powerful unseen force. Love is Light, that enlightens those who give and receive it. Love is gravity, because it makes some people feel attracted to others. Love is power, because it multiplies the best we have, and allows humanity not to be extinguished in their blind selfishness. Love unfolds and reveals. For love we live and die. Love is God and God is Love.

This force explains everything and gives meaning to life. This is the variable that we have ignored for too long, maybe because we are afraid of love because it is the only energy in the universe that man has not learned to drive at will.

To give visibility to love, I made a simple substitution in my most famous equation. If instead of $E = mc2$, we accept that the energy to heal the world can be obtained through love multiplied by the speed of light squared, we arrive at the conclusion that love is the most powerful force there is, because it has no limits.

After the failure of humanity in the use and control of the other forces of the universe that have turned against us, it is urgent that we nourish ourselves with another kind of energy…

If we want our species to survive, if we are to find meaning in life, if we want to save the world and every sentient being that inhabits it, love is the one and only answer.

Perhaps we are not yet ready to make a bomb of love, a device powerful enough to entirely destroy the hate, selfishness and greed that devastate the planet.

However, each individual carries within them a small but powerful generator of love whose energy is waiting to be released.

When we learn to give and receive this universal energy, dear Lieserl, we will have affirmed that love conquers all, is able to transcend everything and anything, because love is the quintessence of life.

I deeply regret not having been able to express what is in my heart, which has quietly beaten for you all my life. Maybe it's too late to apologize, but as time is relative, I need to tell you that I love you and thanks to you I have reached the ultimate answer!"   Your father, Albert Einstein

The Law of True Success

Believe not because some old manuscripts are produced, believe not because it is your national belief, believe not because you have been made to believe from your childhood, but reason the truth out, and after you have analyzed it, then if you find it will do good to one and all, believe it, live up to it and help others live up to it.

The Unknown

Several decades ago, I experienced an out-of-body experience (mind projection). It set me on a spiritual path of meditation, yoga, and the study of religions. I clearly defined my fundamental purpose: Freedom. However, when many years later, I discovered The Code of Life, I learned that meditation is a wrong practice that eventually disorients genes in six brain glands, the same glands that are damaged by the drugs and perpetuated lies (that is the same as believing in a lie), that instead, it must be practiced the mind watching. I also learned that only a few yoga routines are useful: different routines for different people. I also discovered that the entire Eastern spiritual industry, with all its self-appointed teachers and gurus, is but a hoax, a lie based on two useless books of Vedas and Upanishads, which energy level is only 5%, meaning an outright fraud.

I also made a living and had material goals to attain. This combination of the material path and spiritual often made me contemplate material success, causing an inquiry to reside in the back of my mind: is there a rule that can be learned and applied that will allow one to harness material success without losing their spiritual goal of Freedom? Like most people, I tend to believe that material success is measured with money, and the desire for money thwarts inner growth. Yet, in my heart, I was convinced that there must be a formula for True success, and I kept searching for it.

It happened during the production of the Russian-American Investment Symposium when I felt for the first time that I had stumbled on something real. I felt close, yet I couldn't define The Formula of True Success. It was only when I "discovered" Andrew Carnegie that I found it.

Andrew Carnegie helped me realize that only with Love can one grow happy and rich when wealth is created to benefit people and provide modestly for one's dependents, and oneself is a perfect example of how one can find Love and Happiness; Andrew Carnegie is an ideal example of how Love can harmonize Happiness and wealth. Thus, I bow to Andrew Carnegie with gratitude for the supreme gift of the precious treasures of knowledge and imagination through which everyone may ascend into a life of true happiness and riches.

Regarding true success, which means Happiness plus material success, success books are misleading. Authors mention "happiness" many times but never say what happiness means. Also, the concept of Love is absent in these books, and the meaning of Compassion, loving-kindness, acceptance, and true success. Yet, these qualities have made Andrew Carnegie's success different from all other very successful business people. Looking at those who have risen from rags to riches, it appears that the absence of Love created selfish, greedy people apathetic to their poorer brethren, , who made them wealthy.

There is no such thing as the Law of success, nor are there rules that help create wealth. If there were such laws or rules, anyone could create wealth by learning those rules. The Law of success, taught to eager crowds, is a hoax, unaware created in a dream world, the theory that was never proven true. Blinded by the desire for wealth, people believe that studying and closely following examples of those who rose from rags to riches may become equally successful.

Those who have risen from rags to riches could never explain how they did it. Volumes have been written on the subject of how to become rich. However, there is no explanation of the mechanics of the process because there is none. There only are some foggy hints, some common qualities of character, etc., which means nothing because one unique thought makes a great deal of difference.

A never known secret lies in the uniqueness of each emotional-thinking process, in the intensity of related thoughts, in a matchless thought pattern, in the influence and cooperation of the participants, in the timing and circumstances of that time, in the ability to sense a right opportunity, as well as in many other unknowns, which are impossible to describe, never mind – to recreate. The world is changing every instance, and there can be no two sets of the same circumstances or persons separated in time, except for the illusion of similarity created by the mind.

Further down, there is an explanation of the difference between the Law of success and The Law of True Success.

"Nearly twenty years ago," writes Napoleon Hill in Law of success, "I interviewed Mr. Carnegie for the purpose of writing a story about him. During the interview, I asked him to what he attributed his success. With a merry little twinkle in his eyes, he said: "Young man, before I answer your question, will you please define your term 'success'?"

"After waiting until he saw that I was somewhat embarrassed by his request, he continued: "By success, you have reference to my money, have you not?" I assured him that money was the term by which most people measured success, and he then said: "Oh, well, if you wish to know how I got my money - if that is what you call success - I will answer your question by saying that we have a mastermind, etc."

If you paid attention to the above, you would surely notice Carnegie's question, "By success, you have reference to my money, have you not?" This question should have led Hill to ask Carnegie what he, Carnegie, meant by success, but Hill didn't ask the most important of all questions.

All success coaches fell into this cultural trap that made them fall short of recognizing Love's major role in true success, which means Happiness plus material success. Society creates wrong beliefs of success, meaning money, and money meaning true Happiness.

Our society is devoid of Love; without Love, it cannot understand true happiness. Consequently, it fails to recognize that true Success cannot happen without Love and Happiness: "Previous studies have found," writes a Times reporter, "that $75,000 is the earnings tipping point in terms of happiness: Anything above that mark has no long-term effect on happiness, but each dollar below the $75,000 figure decreases happiness. Also, Happiness is directly related to how much money we make. We've known that for a while." Shouldn't the word satisfaction be used here instead of happiness? Resistance is the main reason for such an ignorant attitude bordering on stupidity toward Love and Happiness. Created involuntarily, a subconscious program of Resistance defends all our conscious and subconscious ignorance.

Who was people's teacher in the past, and what did it teach? It was church. Because of a lack of Right knowledge, the church is forever guided by a wrong knowledge that blinds it to Love and Happiness.

Right knowledge also includes knowledge of Love's capability to improve human life and Love's powerful means of solving social problems. Yet, regulated by the government, whether in the US, Russia, or China, the educational system doesn't teach a supreme role of Love in creating a life of Happiness, despite the Right knowledge being freely available. Because society doesn't consider Love and Happiness, it doesn't know what true Success is.

Humanity's life means each person lives in his or her dreamland. Combined, these dreamlands form humanity's dreamland, constituting humanity's subconscious field. The reason for the subconscious to be purged of negativity by transforming the past into Love is to purify the mind of its illusory dreaming, where reality is perceived through a prism of mostly negative conditioning.

Andrew Carnegie is a unique example. Another example is Sam Simon; other people gained the Right knowledge to break through cultural conditioning. However, Andrew Carnegie is an exceptional example. He was brought up with Love. Love shielded Andrew from cultural conditioning and made him preserve a loving mind, which enabled him to live in the land of reality.

All things are perfectly resolved in the pure mind, accessible only by free people. Yet, gracious nature is truly generous with her gifts: it gifted everyone with Love – an extension of Infinite Intelligence in the human world and endowed it with the same ability to resolve all things perfectly. The more loving the mind is, the higher its Intel-Star energy level and the more appropriate your decisions are. The sooner you define your most fundamental purpose that will be harmonious with your inherent abilities, the better.

Do you realize that Love alone can bring Happiness, even without developing fundamental qualities of the character necessary for Success? It can do that because, being our essence, Love contains and, when awakened, "enables" fundamental character qualities necessary to ensure your success. Yet, an irrevocable decision to create a life of happiness, persistence, determination, and unshakable faith in Love is required to develop for Love to become your leader.

Suppose you choose not to transform your past into Love. In that case, you may still guess/decide on your definite purpose, develop your fundamental character qualities, and become materially successful by chance, but you will not know Happiness. Your relationships will suffer, and you will suffer. You will remain unfulfilled no matter how wealthy and famous you may become, for this is the destiny of all achievers who lack Love. When one doesn't know about Love, it is better to suffer a life of the rich rather than the misery of being poor. But even having this kind of choice, what chance do you have to become rich? You may waste your life pursuing riches. Yet, when you know what Love brings, isn't it logical to explore the way of Love?

As it was in Andrew Carnegie's life, Love and Happiness must come first to ensure success is whole –true Success. You may be a plumber and live a life of Happiness, which will be incomparably more beneficial than the life of J. D. Rockefeller, for nothing matters more to the person himself than Happiness, which is an inner state of serenity and Love, dependent on nothing in the outside world.

You may know the story of the president of "an island of refugees in a world of crazy people" – José Mujica, president of Uruguay. Is there any other president in the whole world who would be as nearly honest, open, and happy as Mujica?

With Love, like Carnegie's and Mujica's, you will be rewarded with Happiness – the most precious of all life's gifts. We learn the value of Love and our purpose, what we can do best to benefit others and ourselves, and when led by Love, our intel-Star energy level is high, and our choice is always right.

As Andrew Carnegie demonstrated, Love and Happiness happened to be the main ingredients of true Success, for success without Love and Happiness is nothing but a compromise – a deceiving illusion of success.

The Law of True Success is simple to grasp: Love and Grow Happy and Rich. Andrew Carnegie lived by this Law, and so can you. The secret of the Law lies in the right blend of success's potion ingredients and its intense "cooking" in the fire of imagination and Love. The key to this secret is the Love that will guide you to making the right blend, resulting in "Carnegie's success" of Happiness and abundance.

Without Love, The Law of True Success becomes the so-called Law of success, which is not a law but deception. It neither rules Success nor can it bring Happiness. People, who become successful without Love, come to a life of a troubled rollercoaster of success, disappointment, stress, misery, and so on, often suffering more than an average person.

Most people trying to be successful do not know about the imperative role Love plays in the creation process, and without Love's guidance, this process becomes guessing. If you lack one or more of the fundamental qualities of character or intensity, you may fail if you don't guess the right opportunity, people, and time (for it is all guessing). However, lack of Love will fail your life, for Happiness is the purpose of everyone's life.

The worldly hope men put their hearts upon
Turns ashes, or it prospers and anon,
Like snow on dusty desert's face
Lasting a little hour or two… is gone

Omar Khayyam

Almost a thousand years past, Omar Khayyam has described the destiny of the "successful" that knew no Love. There is no law, rule, or key to material success devoid of Love. A lottery called great material success or the American dream is exclusively a matter of the extremely rare chance, an accident.

It is why only a few accidentally rose from rags to riches, experiencing much suffering, much trouble, using much effort, mercilessly exploiting others, and ending with no Happiness. Every "captain of industry" went through this mill and died a man of greed and deceit. It makes people believe that suffering is a necessary part of success. Wrong! Suffering is inevitable only in the absence of Love. Carnegie's life is best proven in a great rise from rags to riches into an unparalleled success created naturally, honestly, with no suffering.

We are born with a different set of basic tendencies and a 100% Intel-Star energy level – a potential for a successful life of Happiness. The tendencies hint at your talent and what vacation would best be in accord with this talent. Today, neither parents nor teachers can reveal this set of tendencies in a child. Rarely, usually accidentally, is this discovery made, and even less often, the child's talent gets the help to be fully developed. This is the main reason why there are so many unhappy people with what they do in life. However, when a child is brought up with Love, he would have an incomparably better opportunity to create a life of Happiness.

Not everyone is destined to be wealthy, but everyone is potentially destined to be successful in some area of life and be truly happy. Fortunately, there is Love that shields us from mistakes. When Love leads us, we will make no mistake in choosing an occupation that is harmonious with our talent and will contribute to our success: a life of Happiness.

When they realize the outright importance of true Love, an incomparable benefit of Love's guidance, most people will not fail to build a life of Happiness.

To everything, there is a season and a time to every purpose under the heaven.

Wisdom of the universe is hidden within this seemingly obscure line: it accurately describes the law of success. It says there is no need for craving and pushing. All we need to do is accept that we, with our little egos, can do nothing– the Infinite within and without is the only doer.

A man is given a choice of conceiving or not conceiving a thought, idea, or action.
When we decide to act, several important points must be kept in mind to ensure successful results:

1.   We eliminate doubt, cravings, and pushing. I.e., we get our little ego out of the way and let the Infinite

unobstructed to carry on the task. With such an attitude, we see what needs to be done.

2.	We calmly do whatever needs to be done, but there are no cravings for the result. Instead, full attention is given to the process.

It may be called detachment or surrender, but it is also common sense. Every emotion is an abstraction, every doubt – is an impediment, and each thought is a limitation. When a mold of a goal is created with a mechanism of thought and fire of determination – it is bound to materialize. No other thoughts or emotions are necessary. It is determinably conceived, envisioned, and dropped – accomplished in the beholder's mind.

When something is accomplished, it is usually let go to 'live' its own life, only to be helped when help is needed. Much aid may be needed during the project's life, but the project is already accomplished and finished as far as its creator is concerned. In our mind, a goal has already been accomplished. Why worry about having done something that has already been done? But usually, this is not the case. It is difficult for us to believe in something we do not see. What is this Infinite? How can raising the money needed to finance the project be accomplished? It is philosophy; what I need – is hard cash. We move on, pushing an accelerator and applying the brake simultaneously.

But if man's ability to get himself in trouble is limitless, still, the resourcefulness of the Infinite is inexhaustible. A simple and very powerful method, thus, is to be your best and only teacher and release all abstractions, limitations, and impediments to our success in everything we desire to accomplish.

About the Author

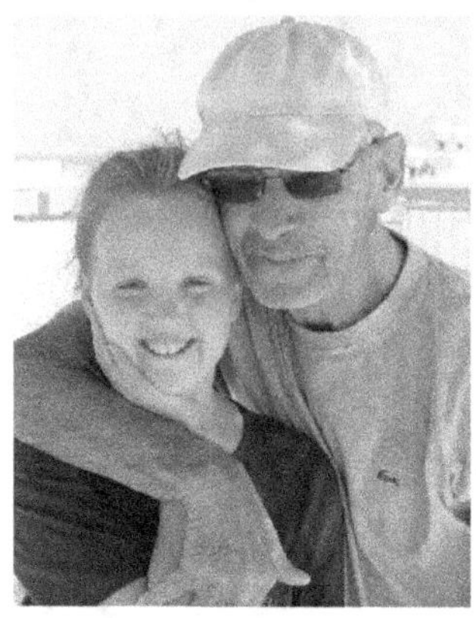

Yuri Spilny was born in Vladivostok, Russia. His life has been varied and unusual. After six years in the Navy School, Yuri decided it was not for him. "When awakening for duty, I was hit with the sudden realization," he said, "Now walk out of here! And I left the Naval Academy just three months before graduation." Yuri then went to Moscow Film School and began a successful career as a documentary filmmaker. Traveling the world, he produced over 70 documentary films on various subjects. Yuri lectured at the University of Economics and Moscow State University on Awareness, Responsibility, and Freedom. He studied comparative religious philosophy and practiced meditation. He created and produced the *Russian-American Investment Symposium* in partnership with the *J. F. Kennedy School of Government, Harvard University*. His company, *USSR Film Service Corporation,* represented the Russian Film Industry in the US, facilitating and producing numerous films, including *Chernobyl, the Final Warning, Inside the KGB,* and *Cops in Russia.*

"I always knew," he says, "that my destiny was to write," and he wrote *The Incredible Adventures of Kitto*, a beautifully illustrated trilogy of fairy tales emphasizing to young readers "every child is born to succeed." His books *Gates of the Dead,* a novel; *Freedom Technique: Path to Awareness and Love; The Lion Moves Alone,* and other books are at Amazon.com. For twenty years, Yuri lived in Sierra Mountains in the heart of Sequoia National Forest, California.

yuri@bookstoejoy.com

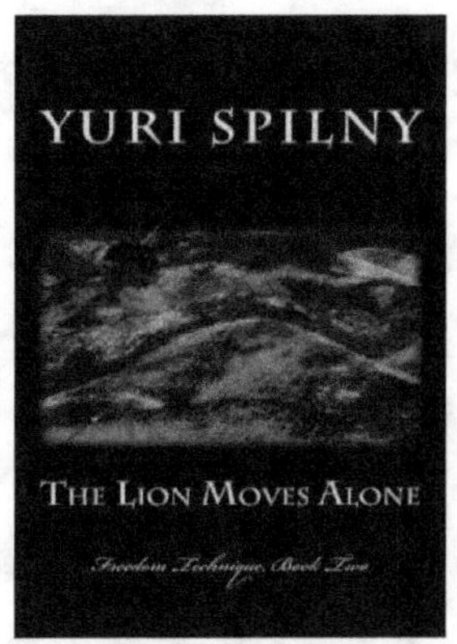

First comes desire, followed by hope, disappointment, and suffering; then comes search. Search discovers Love. With Love comes the simplicity of being in the "now" and joy that melts desires. The mind is educated when your entire past is transformed into Love. When it happens, Love becomes the leader, and the educated, aware mind follows Love's intuitive lead.

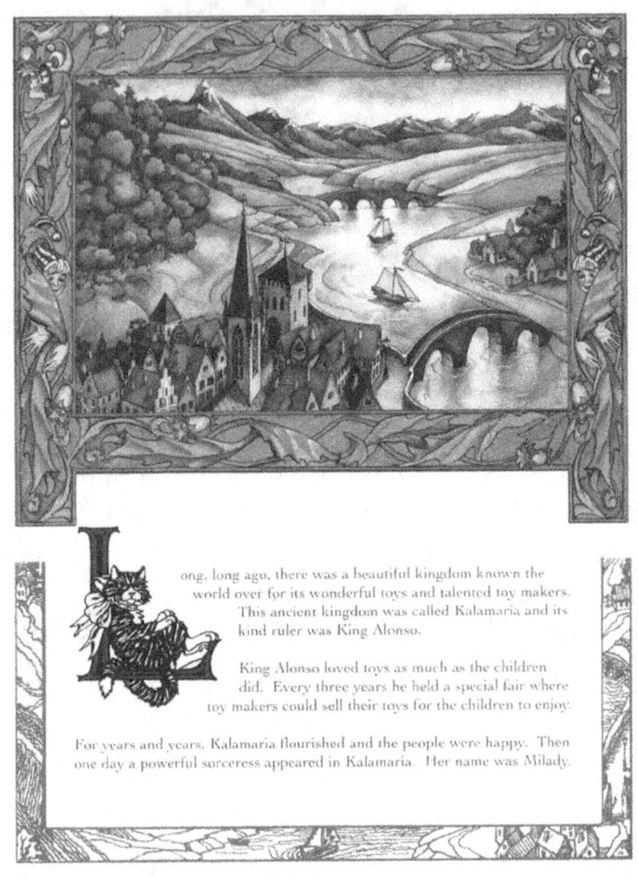

The Incredible Adventures of Kitto

Set of three books (8.5"x 11") with over 80 original illustrations in Full Color

A set of three original books is available at www.bookstoenjoy.com

E-books,are available at Amazon.com

THE MIDWEST BOOK REVIEW

The Incredible Adventures of Kitto
Yuri Spilny
Bookstoenjoy.com
HC1, Box 106, Kernville, CA 93238
yuri@bookstoenjoy.com

Beautifully illustrated with more than eighty original watercolors, "The Incredible Adventures of Kitto" is a wondrous trilogy of fairytale stories that emphasize to their young readers "every child is born to succeed."

Sorceress's Spell (1-892316-00-5) follows ten-year-old Kitto as he incurs the wrath of the wicked Milady. Escaping Milady's powers via a flying dragon and aided by the good Fairy Sambhava, Kitto creates four magical toys which become Kitto's best friends. The Toynapers (01-3) finds Kitto bringing his toys to participate in The Greatest Toy Show on Earth, where Princess Daisy falls in love with them, and her father makes Kitto his royal toy master -- only to see Kitto end up falsely accused of a terrible crime, convicted and imprisoned. River of Fire (02-1) begins with a breathtaking escape for now blind Kitto through the services of his good friend, the flying dragon. Aided by Fairy Sambhava once again, Kitto and his toys travel to the Enchanted River of Fire. Together they encounter and overcome great dangers. Eventually, they reach the Pearl Palace of a terrible wizard and obtain a very special treasure.
A highly recommended fairytale trilogy.

James A. Cox, Editor-in-Chief

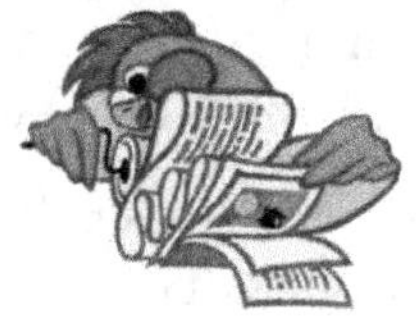

www.ingramcontent.com/pod-product-compliance
Lightning Source LLC
Chambersburg PA
CBHW061336250726

48657CB00004B/1194